PATHWAYS

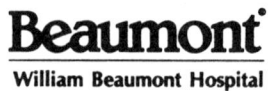

Beaumont
William Beaumont Hospital

William Beaumont Hospital
Speech and Language Pathology Series

MICHAEL I. ROLNICK, PH.D.
Series Editor

Books in this Series

Right Hemisphere Stroke: A Victim Reflects on Rehabilitative Medicine, by Fred K. Johnson, 1990

Pathways: Moving beyond Stroke and Aphasia, by Susan Adair Ewing and Beth Pfalzgraf, 1990

PATHWAYS

MOVING BEYOND STROKE AND APHASIA

SUSAN ADAIR EWING, M.A. CCC
BETH PFALZGRAF, M.A. CCC

WAYNE STATE UNIVERSITY PRESS   DETROIT

Library of Congress Cataloging-in-Publication Data

Ewing, Susan Adair, 1943–
    Pathways : moving beyond stroke and aphasia / Susan Adair Ewing,
Beth Pfalzgraf.
        p. cm. — (William Beaumont Hospital speech and language
pathology series)
    Includes bibliographical references.
    ISBN 0–8143–2074–0 (alk. paper). — ISBN 0–8143–2075–9 (pbk. :
alk. paper)
    1. Aphasia—Case Studies. 2. Cerebrovascular disease—Case
studies. I. Pfalzgraf, Beth, 1955– . II. Title. III. Series.
RC425.E95   1990
616.85'5206—dc20
                                                         90–12148
                                                            CIP

Acknowledgments
    The authors want to thank Dr. Michael Rolnick, series editor and director of
the speech and language pathology department, William Beaumont Hospital,
Royal Oak, Michigan, for his help and encouragement. Special thanks are due to
Dr. Keith Camann, doctor of internal medicine, Lansing, Michigan, who served
as medical consultant.

To the courage of those living with the loss of speech and
language and their families, who took the time
to share their thoughts, feelings, and often painful memories
so that others could learn

Contents

Contents

Preface

Stroke is swift, unexpected, and devastating. In its aftermath are feelings of confusion and fear, as the survivors of this illness and their families begin a long struggle through the various stages of recovery. Most, with little, if any, previous exposure to what a stroke is all about, feel alone, unsure of where to turn for help. Many are afraid this illness means resignation and loss of hope, perhaps not aware that "getting better" is more possible now than ever before.

Today, fortunately, the image of stroke is changing away from the picture of helplessness this illness produced years ago. Recovery from a stroke can and does happen, when not so long ago little could be done. Advances in medical science and rehabilitation techniques have made treatment more effective than ever before. Since awareness about strokes is increasing with more information about prevention, medication, and therapies, support for those affected is more readily available. Indeed, hopeless isolation is no longer the future for the survivors.

In the dictionary the word stroke is defined as "a sudden action or process producing an impact"; in medicine this sudden change refers to a disruption in the flow of blood to brain tissue. There are many different reasons a stroke, or cerebral vascular accident (CVA) occurs, as well as many different kinds of strokes. The areas of the brain a stroke affects depends on where the blood supply was interrupted. When this happens in the language area of the brain, most commonly in the left hemisphere, then aphasia, or loss of communication, is the result. Most of us associate this only with loss of the ability to speak, but "communication" also involves listening, thinking, responding, reading, and writing. Each of these abilities, in varying degrees, is affected for the person who has aphasia. Feelings of isolation after stroke are intensified for those who also experience communication loss. It is difficult enough to figure out who to talk with, let alone try to do this when the very act of communication itself is impaired.

As practicing speech and language pathologists in a private suburban hospital, we work daily to help stroke survivors recover lost communication and to help them learn ways to compensate for their new difficulties. We feel that easy-to-understand information about aphasia written for families and for those working with them is not available, and since we think that everyone should have access to this type of material, we decided to provide it.

In doing so we will discuss more than the "clinical" aspects of this illness. We will illustrate what a stroke and aphasia feel like to those experiencing them: how the person with aphasia still clearly comprehends his environment but has lost the ability to communicate effectively in it and how devastating the effects of this disability are on those struggling to interact and react in a culture where verbal communication is essential. Most of all we will emphasize that progress *is* possible. Over time, although perhaps much too slowly, recovery from this illness does occur, even though some of the residuals of stroke and aphasia may still remain.

To accumulate the information necessary to write such a book, we chose six families to work with us on this project. Actual names have been changed to respect the privacy of the individuals involved. We intentionally chose diverse people so that differing insights from persons of varying ages, sex, and degree of physical impairment and communication ability could be shared. The stroke survivors had two things in common: each had sustained his stroke at least three years ago and each had been treated by a speech and language pathologist because of his aphasia.

First, we asked the families to look at a questionnaire focusing on their observations and feelings about the stroke. Then, after each family had taken time to reflect, we interviewed members one at a time. The stroke survivors were asked about their speech and language difficulties; the family members were asked to think about the changes they made in their lives to adjust to the communication loss. All shared insights about the emotional impact of aphasia. In some cases only a few family members wanted to join in, while in others, extended family members were included, especially if they had played a key role in rehabilitation.

As researchers, we were careful to insure that we did not lace the families' recollections with our perceptions, and we met periodically to share information, to check our accuracy, and to compare and contrast our observations.

Finally, we organized these experiences along with our comments into the stages of recovery we thought were particularly relevant: hospitalization, homecoming, and future plans. In addition, since in our practice we are often asked for clarification about the dynamics of aphasia, we take time to explain this language disorder in the section following our "Homecoming" chapter. We also felt that the emotional adjustments following a stroke were important enough to warrant a chapter of their own, "Psychosocial Issues Related to Stroke and Aphasia."

As we gathered information for this book, we found an interesting phenomenon occurring. When family members met with us and with each other in their homes, they began to talk about the stages of their healing. They shared feelings they had not discussed before and discovered new perspectives as they became able to express what was once too painful or fearful to face. Many said they felt this an invaluable experience for furthering their own growth, growth in the marriage, and growth of the family. This time of sharing helped them to heal, offering an opportunity to continue moving in new directions. The families selected the term we use throughout, "stroke survivor," feeling it gave the most hopeful description of recovery.

And so we begin, having deepened our respect for the individuals and families who have experienced all that we write about. We applaud each of you who have reminded us that bridges to restore communication can indeed be built.

1.

Before the Stroke

In the next six chapters we enter the private lives of six families touched by stroke and aphasia. Each family has shared thoughts, feelings, and details of its experiences during the struggle to recover. Each responded differently to this crisis of stroke according to its own intricate web of family structure, roles, and past experiences.

Before we begin sharing the details of each person's stroke and communication loss we felt it important to share what the stroke survivors' lives were like up until that time. Where were they living? What were the patterns in their particular family? What was important to them and how did they approach problems? By looking at life before the stroke we can better understand how personality might play a role in recovery. As we continue, we can discover the similarities and differences in each person's response to this change.

We do this recognizing that it is impossible to convey a complete picture of all that makes up one person at any given moment in time, for perceptions, attitudes, and experiences merge to create uniqueness. This is one reason why recovery courses can never be fully predicted—there are just too many variables. Conditions are perceived and coped with differently by different personalities. (An additional factor, of course, is physiological—healing time after a stroke varies according to the location, severity, and type of brain injury.)

No path to recovery is the same and none is the "right" one. Every story illustrates that the direction one chooses is influenced partly by the direction from which one has come. To begin, then, let us look backwards—to the start of each path.

Ed

He glanced up at the soft rapping on his door.

"Time to go, Ed."

A quick look at his watch told him it was past 7:30 and long after twilight.

Thousands of hours had been spent in this cluttered office—reading, writing, listening . . . perhaps helping a lost student get back on track. And many other hours had been devoted to more than "just a few" other experiences. While some life paths follow predictability, Ed Collins had traveled a winding one in his sixty-two years. He had written a book in Acapulco, meditated in the desert with Hopi Indians, taught himself seven languages, and led a platoon of men through battle in World War II.

The latch caught softly as he pulled the door closed behind him. Footsteps echoed down the empty hall.

Underlying all this activity was a sense of curiosity so fierce Ed became driven when immersed in a project. The drive was for knowledge—its intensity motivated but also frustrated him when there were no answers. Then he would write, pouring out his feelings, opinions, and theories about life. So far these ideas had been published as a textbook for students and a storybook for children. Ed knew there would be more books.

The exit door swung outward, letting in the neon from the streetlight above.

Although sensitive to others' needs, the price for awareness and understanding was painful, especially when he remembered the atrocities of the war and, lately, his close friend's fight with terminal cancer. Losing him was devastating. Depression had settled, bringing withdrawal into himself as he sorted out his feelings and the future he faced. He was not ready to retire from his tenured position as a professor of psychology at the city university. Status had been hard-won. His unique approach to teaching the subject brought both criticism and applause, but always respect. For it was Ed who "lit fires" in students as he wove his life adventures into his lectures, as he tutored those who needed special attention, or as he banned traditional testing methods in his classes. His love of teaching and the influence he had had on so many students through the years were his inspiration and motivation.

Fumbling with keys in the shadowed garage, Ed turned the lock and spilled his pile of papers on the seat beside him. The

Olds engine caught and he backed from the space bearing his name.

Ed brought his characteristic love and energy to his family relationships. Even though the children were grown he visited whenever possible, delighting in the antics of his grandchildren. Leisure time was filled with activity, sometimes exhausting to those around him, for Ed was always "doing" or "thinking" about something, always conscious of a need to explore. Friendships revolved around the university. Travel centered upon scheduled research projects and weekend trips upstate to the family's mobile home.

Light flowed through the glass panel in the front door, making a bright patch in the snow on the front lawn. Cutting the engine, Ed scooped his papers together. It wasn't too late. Julie would be home from her meeting at church; dinner would be ready. They would share talk about the day, perhaps touch upon unfinished plans for travel and retirement. The bond of their marriage drew closer as the years passed. Struggles to overcome the insecurities of youth had long been put aside. The future held promise of a pathway that would continue to wind in and out of new places.

Betty

The sprawling suburban neighborhood where Betty Dankin had lived since her marriage to Bill eighteen years ago was always at its best at dawn, when dew-topped lawns glistened in peaceful silence. Lately, on mornings like this, having a cup of coffee, a newspaper, and a chance to enjoy her surroundings seemed like a much better choice than facing the congested expressway to work. Still, balancing work, home, and play on days like today was a pleasure to Betty.

She stopped behind the blinking school bus collecting children from the neighborhood. Not many left now . . . most residents were older, having raised their children and started their retirement, winding down careers with the automobile companies in town. Betty herself had spent the last twenty-three years working as an accountant for one of these companies, where it had been her private challenge to make order out of chaos: manipulating numbers, equalizing accounts.

It was after 12:00 before she realized she had fallen behind in her morning work already. Betty swept last week's report aside, grabbed her purse, and headed out for the first of her lunchtime errands. As she paid for the thick fabric ordered last week she wondered if the patterns she designed would look as she had imagined. She had sewed her own wardrobe for so many years it was hard to remember ever buying clothes off the racks. Although work associates wondered where the time and energy came from, Betty found sewing totally engrossing; it released creativity and relaxed her. Sewing, playing the organ, participation in a work golf league—all these filled Betty's life when she wasn't working.

Her mind wandered as she walked back to the office. In all her fifty-one years she had never been at a loss for activities to fill the time; there were so many things to do and see. Yet sometimes she questioned whether there really would be enough time to do it all. Thoughts like these had come more often since the recent and overwhelming loss of her mother. For the first time, Betty had to face the reality of her own mortality, and she longed for the comfort only those facing similar pain could provide. Her sister was too far away, living with her husband in Syracuse, and even though her two brothers lived in town, they rarely saw one another, occupied in lives grown separate with the passing years. Friends were there, a multitude of acquaintances who crammed "living and loving" into many shared activities. But it was only upon her mother's death that she had come to realize—because of her own reluctance to really open up to them—that she didn't feel close to most.

More reports and nine holes of golf demanded her full attention the rest of the afternoon. Heading home was easier this night since rush-hour traffic had passed. Betty looked forward to a hug from Bill, but the house was empty when she opened the door; he wasn't yet through with his own day playing the organ at a nearby funeral home. Passing by the massive organ in their living room reminded her of the days they dated after she took organ lessons from him to improve her skills. They had delighted in this common interest, filling their lives with many hours of music created together.

Bill, twenty years her senior, was now partially retired, stirring ideas within Betty of her own retirement so they could spend more time together. Her concern for Bill had increased recently, spurred by a realization he was developing medical problems. His heart was failing, and his memory was deteriorating more than it should even for his age. Betty shared her worries with her three stepchildren, who had always welcomed her into their lives, and found tremendous support in their mutual concern.

Her hand drifted across the polished mahogany of the organ as her thoughts drifted back to the present. Life was moving ahead to new phases in spite of her reluctance to face some of them. Betty was aware she might have to shoulder more responsibility if Bill's health continued to decline, perhaps making difficult decisions about his long-term care.

She silently blessed her own good health and the inner strength that had always carried her through whatever life stages she had had to face. What was next? For now, she longed for the serenity of morning.

Ted

Mazel tov. Twelve more graduates of Hebrew school. Twelve more ready to pass on the traditions of Jewish culture. Ted Lambert's commitment to his religion began as a child and remained a significant part of his life. Tonight Ted celebrated a graduation made possible, in part, by the enthusiasm and leadership he transmitted to his students.

Religion was not the only arena for this energy. Ted had always exuded confidence through circumstances others found defeating, like the recent failure of his printing business. Years before, Ted's father started the family business, handing the reins to his son shortly after Ted's graduation from college. Financial security followed, giving Ted, his wife, and their four children a chance to enjoy some of the rewards of his success. But a combination of poor location in an aging city and reduced capital eventually forced him into bankruptcy. Ted was forced to sell both his car and home. In spite of the blow he was more angry than discouraged and determined to overcome this financial setback.

Ted hugged the last of the youngsters leaving with parents for homes across the city. As he drove to his own, the sun dipped toward the horizon. Today's training run would be done in darkness. Only one more week stood between training and his first marathon. Emphasis on health and fitness had developed only since 1983, after triple bypass surgery to repair damage done by a lifetime of obesity, heavy smoking, and working too many long hours. Facing life-threatening surgery shocked him into realizing how badly he had abused his body. After surgery the cardiovascular team at the hospital provided the impetus and encouragement for Ted to quit smoking, lose weight, and start to exercise. Used to pushing himself, Ted found a new goal in improving his level of health and fitness through resuming a long-forgotten childhood pleasure—running.

Now, one year later, Ted had kept his promise to change. Feeling as if nothing could stop him, at age forty-eight he was far more goal-oriented than ever before. Renewed energy had carried him through work in many places before he settled at a friend's company, where he was given the freedom to develop a computer sales business. His enthusiasm transferred to his communication, making him a natural salesman. His commitment was to give his best, whether to customer, friend, or family. No matter what it took he demanded near perfection from himself and others.

His marriage had not been excluded from this commitment. Twenty-six years ago, as he and Alice began their life together, Ted shouldered sole responsibility for decision-making and finances, believing he should assume the role of family provider. As events interrupted the flow of their lives, each found this way of relating incompatible with growth. They sought guidance in marital counseling and learned to share roles with one another. Over the years honesty and love had deepened with each new challenge. Now they took pleasure in life together with their family gathered near.

Ted pulled on running socks and stooped to lace his shoes. He could hear his children, now young adults, watching TV in another area of the house. Alice was finishing work brought home from the gift shop. Pulling the door closed behind him he disappeared into the night, footsteps pounding the pavement.

Paula

Paula Sams, unlike Ed and Betty, had only started her career. She was much younger than the others; life's pathway took an unexpected turn when she found herself scaling the corporate ladder at age thirty-two. Not so long ago she had walked into beauty school full of ambition to cut hair; now she walked through the airport security gates heading for Indiana to host the second of two seminars on her schedule this week.

On the plane, Paula checked her day's itinerary and outlined material for her speech. Now supervisor of a three-state sales force for a major cosmetic corporation, she had worked hard to advance through an opportunity that had virtually fallen into her lap. Having been asked to try selling the cosmetics early in her beautician career, she found success and quick advancement in the company.

She paused to look at the scene below as the flight attendant brought coffee. Such an endless world! Row upon row of tiny suburban checkerboard stretching to the horizon. Nothing felt as electric as the realm of possibility before her; Paula viewed responsibility for her own future with the eyes of an optimist, brilliant and eager to make her ideas happen.

Determination and focus were traits that had carried her through a difficult childhood as the oldest of four. Home life had not been easy since her mother had had brain surgery years before to remove a benign tumor. Although she had lost no mental capabilities as a result of the tumor and operation, incredibly, she remained incapacitated for the next nine years due to complications arising from her body's rejection of the plate used to close her skull. Paula had assumed her mother's role, raising her younger sister, Cathy, a preschooler at the time.

Now Cathy would take care of the apartment while she was in Indiana. In a way, Paula continued to be mother to a more grown-up baby sister, who had just moved in with her. Family remained an important part of life. She crossed town to visit her parents and college-bound brother Ted as often as she could manage. And before her recent divorce she and her husband had traveled or taken off for a night on the town many times with her brother John and his wife. She missed those spontaneous moments as much as she missed her house, having just moved her own "home" to the apartment after accepting the finality of her divorce.

The plane bounced through its landing and rolled to a stop at the gate. Briefcase in hand, Paula hailed a cab for the trip into town. She was early and might have time to visit colleagues from the branch office before her speech. If not now, there would be dinner later or tonight's cocktail party kickoff for the new company acquisition.

Paula chose to keep very active, maintaining many friendships and hobbies, but not at the price of living superficially. She had long been intrigued by spiritual issues, making it a point to stay involved in a metaphysical study group. No matter how busy life became, she made time for herself and others. Likewise, Paula was good at facing her problems head-on, as she had had to with her divorce. Her ambition to succeed gave her an ability to tackle situations directly, seeing the positive side in most circumstances. The future held promise of many more opportunities and challenges. How would she face them? With the same sense of confidence she felt today as she raised the microphone to open the meeting.

Tom

Tom Martin warmed up his red Corvette, revving the engine "just for the hell of it." He still loved this car. Driving it brought out the carefree kid in him. The difference was that he now knew when to play and when to stop. Tommy, his fifteen-year-old son, hadn't learned that lesson yet, and it terrified Tom to see the ghost of his own past in Tommy's behavior. Tonight, problems waited at home. Tom had thought long and hard about ways to deal with his son. Could he teach him to be responsible when he had barely learned himself? At eighteen Tom had left high school full of unresolved family and personal conflicts. Searching for something to fill the undefined void he felt, he traveled from place to place, moving on whenever friendships started to deepen and thus require more commitment. Then he met Lee, the "best thing that ever happened to me," and their friendship quickly ripened. For the first time Tom let himself risk enough to care about another, and they married in 1964. His biggest fear now was that Tommy, too, would have to learn as he had, by trying things on his own. But he prayed his son would at least finish school.

Tom's parents had encouraged him to go to college, perhaps to medical school as his older brother had. It wasn't until after his marriage, however, that he developed the self-discipline to stick with a program. When he and Lee moved back to his home state, he entered pharmacy school with new direction and determination. During that time he formed lasting friendships with others in his college fraternity, learning that fun could be mixed with hard work. As he watched his marriage, his friendships, and his school work thrive, Tom at last felt commitment.

After graduation Tom invested in a pharmacy with a partner. Now he was finally reaping some financial benefits after endless student loans. Tom was also committed to leadership in a professional pharmaceutical organization and at church, where he ran the youth group. His leisure activities were watching sports, water skiing, or meeting friends at a bar for happy hour.

In the last year he and Lee had spent many hours deliberating about raising their kids. Up to now, his wife had taken major responsibility while Tom was in school or occupied with starting his business. The kids needed him more. Concerned that he would lose those who most needed him, Tom had promised to cut back on long work and play hours.

Today he was leaving work early—it was only 4:00. Rolling up the driveway, Tom stopped short of the garage where his daughter Stacey was just putting her bike away. At thirteen, she was such a contrast to Tommy, an honor student in junior high involved in several school activities. So responsible in contrast to Tommy, and yet he was sure she, too, needed more attention. They winked and grinned at each other as he walked toward the porch. It would be so easy to keep going, perhaps pitch softballs to Stacey in the backyard. But if Tom had learned anything at all it was that confrontation, not avoidance, solved problems. Maybe he didn't know exactly *what* to say to Tommy tonight, exactly how to help his son feel confidence and love, but nothing imaginable could make him stop trying.

Carl

6:30 and a buzzing alarm sent serenity flying and Carl Wilson to the shower. What savage law of nature dictated Monday mornings would never get easier, even after sixty-one years of them? As much as he loved his work he relished Sundays like yesterday, spent on his farm upstate where Carl was raising seven horses. Just he and Eileen went now that the kids were grown. Before too long they planned on selling the house and moving north permanently.

Looping his tie about his collar, Carl vaguely wondered what retiring from the company would be like. Twenty years ago he founded and now presided over his own engineering business. The company was doing well, although the early years had presented some struggles. Seventy-hour weeks were the rule. Independence had been the attraction initially; he enjoyed the freedom to make his own decisions and control the development of the business.

In fact the need to control was an issue in all aspects of Carl's life. While some do so in an offensive and overbearing manner, Carl preferred to be firm but flexible in his interactions with others. Family and friends found him exceptionally open. He always intended to have a ready ear to listen or a shoulder to lean on, yet wouldn't withhold suggestion or advice.

In the kitchen Eileen had toast and coffee waiting. The two compared schedules to plan the day. She was cleaning the house this morning, lunching with friends, volunteering a few hours at the hospital in the afternoon, and perhaps shopping before fixing supper. He was meeting with a client in the morning, going over blueprints later, and making calls to negotiate a new contract. He would be home for dinner at 7:30. Mornings and evenings were spent together whenever they could. Theirs was a close, loving marriage, and a traditional one, with Carl the financial supporter and decision-maker. Communication in the family was unusually open. Besides their planning sessions about schedules and events, Carl and Eileen relied heavily on communication of feelings, describing one another as "the closest of friends." Carl loved to exercise his role as husband, provider, and father, perhaps overprotecting in an attempt to shelter his family from adversity.

Yet "adversity" had not been much a part of the Wilson household; their life seemed nearly ideal most of the time. Their four children, Carl Jr., a son from Carl's previous marriage, and daughters Kristen, Susan, and Marsha, were now making homes of their own. With the children gone, Carl and Eileen found that their life together had become a second honeymoon. Though they had always been close, they now felt a new excitement in the relationship. Eileen was free to travel with Carl on business trips or just for fun, to meet new people and see new places. Both loved to socialize, chatting with friends and strangers alike. Perhaps more than for any others in this book, life flowed along easily for them, uncomplicated by adversity. Tomorrows were bright, looking simply like better versions of today.

Conclusion

These are but brief glimpses into the past. The point at which we left each story marks the ending of a time of stability and the beginning of a time of change. It is the point at which pathways turned sharply: Ed and Ted had sudden brain hemorrhages, Carl and Betty had strokes after surgery, Paula became ill because of a congenital abnormality, and Tom suffered a stroke of unknown origin.

What actually happened when each became ill and how did family members respond to the emergency? What filled the patients' days in the hospital and how did the families manage a life at home? All share their experiences in the next chapter, which recounts the earliest stage in the illness.

As the stories continue, it is clear how the pasts and personalities of the stroke survivors and their families impacted on the paths they chose to take.

2.

Hospitalization

The word "hospital" originally denoted a house or inn—a place of shelter where weary travelers could come for "hospitality." Later, the term was used to denote a charitable institution that cared for the aged and infirm. Today it is a place we go when in need of medical and/or surgical treatment—a place that continues, as the word originally implied, to "care for" others. We like to know such a haven exists, yet we have ambivalent feelings about being "cared for," as it means a necessary relinquishing of control. Detaching oneself from the outside world and giving up comfortable roles and routines can prompt much anxiety and confusion, especially when one is simultaneously concerned about one's health. Robert Murphy (1987), an anthropology professor at Columbia University who suddenly had to count himself among the disabled, writes about his reactions to illness and disability in *The Body Silent*. He considers a hospital a "physical and social cocoon," adding that hospitalization makes those who are forced to enter lose their freedom of choice. In order to survive, a patient must be subservient to the hospital system; the "good" patient and family member are those who conform to the carefully planned hospital rules and regulations.

For some of our families the stroke was their first encounter with serious illness. They were scared and confused about the illness itself, and while they needed help and were well "cared for," it took time to adjust to a large, somewhat impersonal facility and to understand their emotional responses to this new situation. All initially went to the emergency ward where diagnosis and a decision about treatment could be made. In some instances, life-saving brain surgery (craniotomy) was recommended; in others, the patient was placed in intensive care or admitted to a medical floor to be monitored. If their care began in the intensive care unit, the next step might be to the "step down" area in the hospital where the ratio of staff to patient was lower before going to a regular medical floor. Each of these six stroke survivors was eventually transferred to a rehabilitation unit within the hospital where speech and language pathology, occupational therapy, and physical therapy continued at a more intensive pace than on the medical floor. (Not all stroke survivors require continued care in a rehabilitation facility; some with aphasia but without a remaining weakness on the right side (right hemiparesis) are discharged when their medical condition stabilizes, while others still acutely ill may initially require specialized care in a nursing home.)

These families had a variety of memories of their hospital stay. Each individual struggled in his own way to "get through" the first stage of illness, learning as much as possible about this sudden disruption in his life and how to cope with the dramatic changes in his responsibilities. Most recall this as the first of many times they were called upon to make decisions alone because one family member was too sick to understand or even to show concern about the situation. What helped them through this period and what might have made their days as a patient or family member easier? Their insights should prove useful for those facing hospitalization and to all those who may see the crisis of major illness at work.

Ed

Ed Collins's memories of the events the day his stroke occurred are vivid but selective and faulty. On January 28, 1985, he was in his office at the university, as usual, meeting with a professor. Later in the morning he also met with a book salesman but has no recollection of the appointment. During this meeting Ed suddenly felt so ill he had to excuse himself. Shortly after, he walked the two blocks to his car, not recognizing familiar passing students, and drove himself home. Ed repeatedly says he recalls "snow everywhere" that day but there was no snowstorm. His wife believes he may have had trouble walking to his car because he was weak and somehow associated this with the cover of snow already on the ground. This association is what he stored in his memory.

Julie heard the turn of the key in the lock shortly after 1:00, surprised to see her husband enter the house so much earlier than usual. She was talking with her daughter and grandson, who were visiting at the time. When she questioned Ed, who was bending over holding his stomach, he answered, "I'm very sick, I have to go to the bathroom." Then he went to bed, telling his wife, "I'll be all right, just let me lie very still."

Julie quickly became aware of Ed's confusion when she tried talking with him as he lay in bed. He recognized her and looked normal, but he could not respond to her questions. Looking out the window, she saw that he had parked the car in front of the neighbor's home, not theirs, and that the front end was smashed. Afraid that Ed had had a car accident and was in shock, she called an ambulance.

By 4:00 that afternoon Ed had been admitted to the emergency ward at the hospital. Over the next few hours Julie was allowed to see her husband only once. She still did not realize what the medical diagnosis was and to this day remains grateful for the help of a friend working in the hospital, who intermittently checked Ed and brought her news of his condition. Julie did not hear from her doctor that her husband had had a stroke until 4:00 A.M. the morning after admission.

Ed was admitted to a regular medical floor. His stroke had been caused by a hemorrhage, or ruptured blood vessel bleeding into brain tissues. The nausea and vomiting he experienced are commonly associated with brain hemorrhage. In his case this occurred in the parietal lobe of the left hemisphere. When such bleeding occurs, surgery is sometimes necessary to relieve pressure, but in Ed's case the bleeding stopped by itself, and the blood formed a hematoma—much as it does when other parts of the body are "bruised." (A hematoma is a mass of blood, usually clotted and confined to a space, caused by a break in a blood vessel.) These brain tissues have not had the oxygen supply abruptly cut off—rather, the injury to brain tissue is a direct result of the blood itself, of increased intracranial pressure, and of reduced oxygen supply.

Ed became increasingly lethargic but did not lose consciousness. He roused when he heard others talking but had a severe receptive and expressive aphasia by the next day. Communication of any reliability was not possible as he was unable to respond to simple yes or no questions, read, write, or speak. Weakness in both his right arm and leg prevented some movements, and visual field examination revealed a right homonymous hemianopsia (reduced visual field on the right side). He stayed on the regular medical floor for seventeen days, until his condition was stable, and then he was transferred to the rehabilitation unit for intensive treatment.

The emotional effect on Julie was devastating at first. "I did very well when I was with someone but cried most of the rest of the time for the first week." After that time she realized that life had changed, that previous routines were not going to work. Ed was not there as before to consult with or to do the things for her at home she did not want to do. Julie resolved her emotional need to include Ed in their decisions in a unique way by taking papers that came in the mail to his hospital bed and reading them aloud as many as five or six times. She realized Ed couldn't understand most of what she was saying, yet by reading slowly and repetitively she helped herself comprehend unfamiliar information. She felt closer to her husband and developed a sense that he was helping her make a mutual decision—she was not alone.

Julie realizes now she knew very little about stroke. Interestingly, she had thought at one time, when both Ed's parents had had strokes, that she knew a great deal. In an effort to educate herself, Julie began to read. Friends sent journal articles and hospital staff gave her material to better understand strokes. Julie found learning through reading to be extremely beneficial.

From the beginning of Ed's illness, she found contact and interaction with his workplace, the university, necessary, but the communication was poor. Initially, Julie needed specific direction about work-related things that should be taken care of. Making decisions about Ed's work was difficult for two reasons: Julie had not had prior involvement in his work, and she was now emotionally exhausted. Communication from the university was more complicated because they knew little about stroke and certainly didn't realize Julie needed direction. As she reflects back upon this early time, Julie thinks a written outline from the university listing just what needed attention and how to go about it would have been helpful.

During the early part of Ed's hospitalization Julie was frightened, not knowing what to do to help. She wanted more information from his physician and frequently left notes on Ed's chart but was frustrated when no response was returned, making her feel alienated from active involvement with her husband's care. Looking back, she realizes his doctor checked Ed daily, and that he would have notified her should anything need to have been changed. She feels absolute confidence in his physician, but it took her several months to develop the patience and faith that everything had been done. She was really reaching out to anyone, hoping they could "make things better," feeling as many do the loneliness of dealing with the illness of a loved one.

Ed has no memories of the first three weeks. He recalls parts of the day the stroke occurred, then remembers bits and pieces of experiences during his month in the rehabilitation unit. Because of increased pressure in the brain from the hemorrhage, more of his brain tissue was affected and a broader range of his behavior changed. Thus, Ed was very confused at first, a confusion compounded by the severity of the communication loss. He was not able to understand directions easily. Such selective memories and limited associations often cause the stroke survivor to have a distorted view of past experiences.

Spouses and family members are also living through the initial crisis with differing perceptions colored by the effects of shock and denial of the illness. In later months our families stated how important it was to communicate what these differing perceptions and experiences were for each person. It was helpful later to "fill in" missing information for the stroke survivor as well. While discussing information for this book Ed and Julie found such an opportunity with one another.

Ed associated the structure of the rehabilitation unit with his past experiences as a soldier wounded by shrapnel in World War II, possibly because it was the only other time in his life he had been so sick and paralyzed. His memories were triggered by the similarity of his shared hospital room with bunk bed barracks, of community dining in a mess hall, and of the daily routine with his regimented schedule in the service. This association triggered so many memories that Ed vacillated between awareness of his present environment and recollections of the war. Because these memories were painful and often filled with fear, this added to his anxiety, making most interactions with others very confusing for him. But Ed also remembers a few times when staff members spent extra time with him. In these moments, such as when his speech and language pathologist read to him from one of his own books, and when a nurse stayed in his room a bit longer than she needed to, his anxieties lessened.

When preparations began for discharge, Ed went home on weekend passes twice. Although eager to leave the sterile environment, long before the weekend ended he was ready to go back to the hospital, longing for its security and predictability. Julie, on the other hand, felt adequately prepared by the conferences she attended with staff, so she looked forward to his return home. Finally, on March 15, 1985, they left the hospital together for the last time.

Betty

The first major medical complication of Betty Dankin's adult life started during a routine physical examination, when her physician detected a suspected cancerous growth on her left lung. Since it was in the early stages, her prognosis was excellent. She was scheduled for immediate surgery, a lobectomy, to remove the growth. Apprehensive but ready to "get on with it" so she could get back to work, Betty did not sleep the night of her admission to the hospital. She was shaken both by the death of her roommate and by the noise and confusion of the medical floor. Following surgery, which started at 8:00 A.M., and what her husband's children describe as a "seemingly endless day," Betty experienced an embolic cerebral vascular accident (CVA), which affected the left parietal lobe of her brain. An embolus such as Betty had can travel to the brain, depriving brain tissue of the necessary supply of blood and oxygen long enough to cause permanent damage. (Occlusive strokes like Betty's, caused by a thrombus (blood clot) or embolus (traveling blood clot) make up 75 percent of all strokes.)

There would have been no way to predict the possibility of this stroke following her routine surgery to remove the growth on her left lung. By the time of Betty's stroke, her family had left the hospital for the night. Shocked and full of questions and concerns, they would have appreciated a personal phone call from the attending physician; instead, a staff person with limited knowledge of stroke and its implications called, leaving them upset and bewildered with many unanswered questions.

Betty awakened in pain from surgery, feeling completely "out of it!" Her first contact was with a hospital attendant who asked her to "hop on the gurney" to take her to the lab for the first of many medical tests. She fell when she tried to get on the cart and she next slowly realized that her entire right side was paralyzed. Amidst the confusion that ensued came the first recognition that "something dreadful had happened—I could not walk." Feeling alone and helpless, she started to cry, thinking, "I am now completely out of control about everything that is to be done to me." Betty's memory of these events is clear and shows more awareness at this early stage about her stroke than many have.

Speech, occupational, and physical therapy started immediately. During bedside sessions her speech and language pathologist asked her to name the pictures of food that she presented, but she could only indicate that she "didn't like the vegetables." With this type of communicative loss, Betty's difficulty was not in understanding others, but in the ability to retrieve and say the words she wanted. She could not correctly identify her body parts as she listened to her speech and language pathologist say each word; she knew she was hearing the names of them, but Betty kept mixing them up. The family remembers most of her initial attempts at speech as sounding "garbled and full of swear words." Betty was aware she was swearing; she felt both ashamed and powerless to control her response. Aware too that the rest of her speech sounded funny, she tried in vain to find the right words.

At first Betty's vision was fuzzy, no longer corrected by her glasses. She, like Ed, had a right homonymous hemianopsia, which reduced her visual field on her affected right side. A frustration she remembers while on the medical floor was that the staff kept putting her telephone and hospital stand on the side she could neither reach nor see very well, and because her communication was too limited to explain, her family had to remind the staff each time they visited.

One memory that stands out during her stay on the medical floor is the sudden awareness of movement in her right foot without any means to communicate this momentous event. The staff, mistaking her excitement for a medical problem, called her doctor. When he arrived, expecting further medical complications, he was instead greeted by Betty proudly wiggling her right foot. "It was the first moment I felt any hope of recovery."

Betty spent three weeks on the medical floor before her transfer to the rehabilitation unit, where she would spend two months. This new floor felt "like the army"; the pace seemed so rapid in her "slowed-down world." She was still confined to a wheelchair but now could speak short phrases and begin, with the aid of her occupational therapist, to relearn to care for herself using only her left hand. Brushing her hair and teeth, washing—all seemed to take forever. Mealtimes in the dining room were especially chaotic, mostly due to the presence of two individuals who had experienced head injuries in automobile accidents. Unlike persons with stroke and aphasia, those with a head injury have diffuse injury affecting all areas of their brain. Because of this difference, their behavior is often erratic and frightening to those who have had a stroke, who are much more aware of their own actions and responses.

Many painful memories unfold as Betty recalls her time on the rehabilitation floor—a major one is her feeling that "there was no personal interaction with the staff." Two staff members do stand out because of their willingness to treat her as "something other than a number on a sheet." One night, unable to sleep and full of emotional pain, she remembers a nurse's aide coming to her room and holding her as she cried. Nothing was said, but that human contact was not forgotten. Another lasting memory was her first shower. She was lifted into the shower stall—wheelchair and all—by a wonderful nurse who "just let the water run all over me": a glorious change from the daily hospital sponge baths.

Betty felt overwhelmed with the never-ending medical tests, having no idea why they were necessary. When she asked, the only response was, "Your doctor ordered them." Even though aphasia limited her communication, she wanted to be part of the medical conferences.

Betty's first visit home was Christmas Day, a month after her stroke. "It was wonderful to be out of the hospital, but frightening! I cried all day. It was exasperating to try to move in my house in a wheelchair!" The entire family was there but they seemed noisier than usual. Betty's aphasia caused her to have reduced tolerance for noise; she was seemingly unable to block out other sounds in the room to focus on what she needed to hear, almost as if several radios were all tuned to different stations. "I was more tired than I had ever felt in my life and so angry I couldn't talk." When she returned to the rehabilitation unit later that night, she felt "completely cut off from the outside world. I couldn't even dial the numbers on my phone correctly because I couldn't remember them long enough to push them in." Betty's job required her to use numbers daily; now she could not add or subtract, and when she was excited or tired—which seemed almost continuously—she was not able to speak.

Eventually Betty attained enough skill to take care of her daily needs and return home. She could walk, no longer confined to a wheelchair. Feeling fully ready or not, Betty went home for good in February, 1983, with a schedule to begin intensive outpatient rehabilitation three days a week.

Ted

In October, 1984, when Ted Lambert arrived home after a regular training run in preparation for his first marathon, he had a bad headache and garbled speech. Only his daughter Susie was home. Frightened by thoughts of what could be wrong (she had already faced the impact of his heart attack just last year), she phoned her mother at work. Alice, Ted's wife, somehow sensed this might be a stroke. "I had someone from work drive me home and when I saw Ted I knew we needed to get to the hospital immediately. I called an ambulance and went to the emergency room." Ted's diagnosis was "spontaneous left temporal intercerebral hematoma" as a result of an arteriovenous malformation (AVM); a medical resident examined Ted and advised immediate surgery as the only way to relieve the pressure from the bleeding in his brain. (An AVM is a congenital abnormality in which the arteries and veins become weakened with age, causing bleeding or hemorhage. Symptoms, as a rule, do not appear until after the third decade of life. Only 1 percent of all strokes are a result of an AVM.)

Ted's abnormality could not have been diagnosed earlier since this headache was his first symptom. Upon hearing the diagnosis, Alice felt a mixture of emotions: "I at once felt deep love, great fear, anger, resentment, and hope." She called a friend to sit with her during the agonizing six hours of surgery. Afterwards, she was frightened by the doctor's words: "Mr. Lambert will never be the same." Although she realized surgery was life-threatening, she had no idea exactly what those words, "never be the same," might mean. Professionals dealing with strokes must not forget the impact of their words on a family in crisis. Understandably, the surgeon, who must react immediately to the medical need, must be most concerned with his patient and often cannot take time to talk to the family. Some hospitals are now responding to such a need by using a patient advocate to assist the family as they deal with a medical emergency.

During surgery, Alice would have appreciated a place where she could have talked privately with her children. Instead, she spent the next five days in a congested intensive care waiting room since Ted had a second surgery thirty-six hours later. She had medical questions that went unanswered because she could find no one to ask and felt overwhelmed with responsibility, thinking, "I am much too young to live with this." After the initial crisis was over, Alice began a journal to record events, thoughts, and reactions. Later her journal served as a resource to help Ted, who remembers nothing.

Ted spent five days in intensive care, then went to the "step down" floor, where he remained one week before his admission to the rehabilitation unit. Alice's memories are vague about this period except, "I was always tired!" Fragments of questions, concerns, and events are all stored in her memory without sequential order. She remembers how crazy it seemed making a decision about what to do with half a head of Ted's hair since he had been shaved for the surgery, and how dismayed the family was seeing Ted hooked up to so many machines with his head bandaged after the surgery. She explains that one night she hired a private nurse so she could go home to sleep, only to find out the next day that the nurse watched television while Ted's hospital roommate took care of him.

Ted, too, was confused after the surgery. One night during an attempt to get out of bed to go to the bathroom he ended up on the floor. After this, the nurses were forced to strap him in bed for his own protection and that of others. Since they were unable to make Ted understand the logic behind this decision, Alice spent more nights at the hospital so she wouldn't worry and Ted wouldn't hurt himself again.

She has other memories of the shocking changes in Ted during those first few weeks in the hospital. As she looked at her husband, he seemed like an old man—very much the way his own father had looked before his death from cancer a few years before. When she listened to him, his speech was meaningless, filled with the only clear word he could use, "labels." Ted continued to try to talk, but few words made any sense; he was frustrated because he couldn't "hear" the defects of his speech and was convinced he must be fine. Surprisingly, Alice was able to understand quite often what he was trying to say by his inflections and gestures, though to others communication with Ted was like a game of charades. Alice struggled to understand what had happened to Ted's ability to communicate. Although she understood his diagnosis was "aphasia," she wanted information about this condition in order to relate to him better. The speech and language pathologist's terminology in explaining aphasia was of little help.

While Alice spent most of her time at the hospital, their children ran the house. Each of them reacted in his own unique ways to this new family crisis, but all recall the intensity of their pain as they watched their father's struggle. Susie associated hospitals with death and the dying so she didn't want to see him. Her grades suffered and she had trouble concentrating in school and resisted talking to anyone about her distress because she didn't know what to say. Sid felt numb but knew that as the oldest he had to take the lead in maintaining the house and watching out for the others. As he saw his father improving, he was finally able to release some of the emotions that at first he felt he shouldn't express. Sid was going through a difficult period in his own life, needing to make some important decisions about his future, and he missed his dad's usual counsel. He wondered if he would ever hear his father's voice again, for now it sounded so different. He hated the hospital and thought the staff talked to his father like a child. In turn, Darrin and Allen resented well-meaning gestures of family friends who tried telling them how to behave because of illness. They felt others were judging them as irresponsible because they were continuing to lead their lives as always, trying to cope the best they knew how with limited understanding of the total implications of stroke and aphasia.

Ted spent four weeks in the hospital rehabilitation unit, but has only partial memories of this time. Mostly he recalls his total dependence on Alice, the one stable element in his confused world. He needed to feel her presence before he could drift off to sleep at night and when others came to relieve her, he was nervous until she returned. Alice repeated daily the story of why he was in the hospital as Ted couldn't seem to understand the reason for seeing an occupational therapist, a speech and language pathologist, and a physical therapist. The therapists expected him to "*push*" for recovery, "but why?" Because communication was meaningless he needed someone who had "kind eyes," he said, then he would work harder. Ted appreciated the explanations of the therapists—even though he couldn't remember from day to day what they had said—but their words made him feel included. He was offered a newspaper once and realized he couldn't read a word; at the time he didn't think this was particularly unusual. He also wore his wristwatch, yet had no idea about the time. These and other incidents made it seem as if he were "floating" through his hospital stay. Most likely Ted was experiencing euphoria as a result of the brain injury; euphoria is a phenomenon making individuals, especially those with injury to the posterior area of the brain, or with a great deal of cerebral edema (brain swelling), unaware of the total implications of the trauma.

Ted remembers, "I was always hungry but food smelled awful." No one had explained that the steroids prescribed to reduce his brain swelling could have the side effect of insatiable hunger. He became discouraged over getting fat again since he had worked so hard to lose weight following his heart surgery. While in rehabilitation Ted was able to memorize his home phone number to call his family. (Because Ted's speech was relatively fluent and he had little awareness of the extent of his communication errors, he did not have the fear many aphasic persons have about using the phone.) Once he learned to dial, he called home continually, having no memory of his previous call or any concept of lapsed time. On one occasion he was so hungry he called home and told his family "to bring food because they just aren't going to feed me again!" He was asked to order from the hospital menu but he couldn't say the right words or read the menu, although he was able to gesture enough at times so the staff could figure out what he wanted. At one point he let Alice know how good Chinese food would taste by pushing his eyelids upward.

Each Saturday while in rehabilitation Ted went home for the day. While this was good preparation for eventual discharge, Alice had no idea what to do with him and found herself watching him constantly, fearing he would fall and hurt himself. Ted says: "All I wanted to do was sleep. I didn't feel a part of anything." Finally he went home for good on November 29, 1984: still confused and scheduled for intensive rehabilitation.

Paula

On September 1, 1982, Paula Sams was wheeled down a hospital corridor into the operating room for the first of two craniotomies to remove an AVM from her brain. Her journey to get to this stage in her illness had been so much longer than those of the others.

Three years before, as she and her mother drove to a nearby town on one of Paula's business trips, she began to get one of the headaches she had recently begun to have so often. This time she was barely able to pull the car off the highway as lights flashed before her eyes and dizziness and nausea overcame her. Both realized the symptoms now meant something was seriously wrong.

Terrified that she might be developing a brain tumor as her mother had, Paula consulted a neurosurgeon. It took three months, but his final diagnosis indicated an arteriovenous malformation in the left basal ganglia, an area of the brain too close to vital life-sustaining centers to risk surgical removal. There was nothing the neurosurgeon could do; eventually Paula would die from this illness. Drawing on her strength and determination, Paula began what was to be a three-year search for help. There was no sudden stroke like the others in this book. As her symptoms became worse she started radiation treatments in an experimental effort to shrink the mass of veins and arteries from the AVM. It was unsuccessful. Weakness in her right side, especially in her arm, appeared. Her ability to verbally communicate, a skill so vital in her work, began to slowly deteriorate. When Paula could no longer write her sales reports and speak fluently, she took a medical leave, confining herself in her apartment, where she received occasional help from her parents.

When her diagnosis was first made in December, 1979, she had been relieved, despite the gravity of her condition, to be able to move from a time of uncertainty toward facing her illness. Living in fear of bad news felt far more emotionally crippling than confronting and dealing with the bad news itself. Although the emotional energy from her forceful personality carried her through a period of time during which she consulted other neurosurgeons, when the news continued to be discouraging her feelings of relief diminished, leaving her frightened and hopeless.

Eventually, Paula's physical pain became intolerable. At first she took Percodan to manage the headaches, arm, and neck pain. When this no longer controlled it she began injections of Demerol. She started having seizures (see "Associated Health Problems" in Chapter 3 for further explanation of seizures) of increasing severity and by March, 1982, needed constant supervision. Her parents began taking turns staying with her, alternating twenty-four hour shifts. Paula was confined to a hospital bed in the living room of her apartment, where she required Demerol injections every three hours to control the pain. (She even remembers desperately asking the paperboy to give her the injection one day when she was unable to hold the syringe herself.) Her seizures increased to five or more per day. Although her neurosurgeon was reluctant to continue Paula's pain prescriptions because of the dangers of addiction and possible liver damage, her mother remembers begging him to continue, struggling to explain the heartbreak of living with her daughter's suffering.

Paula's memories of this time are vague. Because of her constant medicated state, she was confused about daily events. One memory stands clear, however; she knew she no longer wanted to live with suffering and entertained thoughts of suicide. Paula knew she had no way of taking her own life by herself so she discussed it with a close girlfriend and then with her brother. Both clearly understood her pain yet could not imagine bearing the responsibility of her death. Today, Paula is relieved that she made it through this emotional period, allowing opportunity for what couldn't be imagined at the time—a future full of healing and hope.

In August, 1982, Paula's neurosurgeon made yet another referral, and, after more tests and examinations, this new doctor told her family words they had longed to hear—he was willing to perform the surgery.

Paula listened to her physician explain the risks to her family. The procedure itself was life-threatening. Operating that deeply into the brain meant certain brain damage—the extent of which could not be predicted—and it was certain that her right arm and leg would be paralyzed. Her ability to communicate could be affected. Although she accepted most of these risks, feeling that there was no alternative, she confided to her family that she no longer wanted to live if she lost her ability to communicate.

At home, Paula prepared further for surgery. She made tape recordings of her own voice giving words of encouragement and left instructions that this tape be played constantly at her bedside in the hospital after the operation. She became ready for hospital admission with a feeling of acceptance for either possibility—recovery or death.

The first craniotomy lasted fifteen hours. Paula remained in intensive care for the week between surgeries; her mother remembers her "talking without making any sense." The second craniotomy progressed similarly, without complications.

Her youngest brother, Ted, remembers seeing her shortly after surgery. Painfully, he gazed at her swollen head while she lay in her hospital bed. Able to do little else, he masssaged her right leg, which had little feeling in it, as he reminded her, "I love you." When Paula spoke to return Ted's caring words, it was not "I love you, too," she uttered, but "meatballs." The enormity of all Paula had lost—even basic communication—frightened him. Her brother John also visited with his wife and was shocked when he saw what seemed to be a completely different person. Paula stared vacantly at him with "eyes that looked through me." He cried openly with his wife afterwards, a part of him wondering if Paula was really better off alive.

Paula's first memories after surgery were spiritual. It is hard for her to relate her feelings about this powerful moment, since she is aware that most people respond with skepticism. Nonetheless, she has found energy and motivation from this personal memory that has helped time and again to sustain her through despairing moments. In this experience Paula floated away from her body when she was in surgery to a place "filled with soothing light." The spirit of a monk then took her before God. Although she wanted to stay, God told her that it was not time for her death, that there were further things for her to accomplish in her life. (When Paula shared this memory with her family as we gathered information for this book, she learned for the first time that her father had picked up a pamphlet from the waiting room table the day before her surgery. This pamphlet told the story of a celebrated friar who helped those suffering illness. He offered a silent prayer for his daughter, never knowing this was the same monk who later appeared in her vision.)

First memories for the family during this time of hospitalization were filled with shock over the loss of personality as a "dazed" Paula stared at them with no sign that she recognized anyone. Since she was no longer able to speak, they guessed at her feelings by watching her facial expressions. But Paula had severe comprehension problems as well. Little verbal information was understood and most of her awareness was based on what she touched, saw, or smelled. With communication gone it was difficult for the family, already emotionally exhausted, to continue coping without getting reassurance from Paula that they were doing the right things for her.

When she was medically stable, Paula was transferred to another hospital to begin rehabilitation. The day she left was terrifying. She saw the ambulance and her family gathered around her but she recognized none of them. Prevented by her aphasia from understanding, Paula thought something terrible was about to happen. Even after starting treatment in this new hospital she was scared and confused as to what was happening to her. It is here that her memories begin to emerge with clarity. She felt inadequately informed about her condition, yet realizes now that her comprehension difficulties contributed to a lack of awareness of what health care professionals may have told her at the time.

Being a patient in the rehabilitation unit was difficult. Since she was depressed about her condition she found it hard to go to the dining room where she was surrounded by others who were also ill. She was angry that she couldn't say what she wanted. There were no words, and she didn't know what she was supposed to do, while at the same time she was not fully aware of her own lack of understanding. Part of her anger was from frustration that others were "causing confusion." "I think I was crying a lot but it might have been on the inside."

She feels she "grinned" most of the time outwardly in an effort to fit into a world that was now foreign to her. When doctors made rounds she wondered why they were there. Insight was limited since the lack of comprehension made verbal explanations from others of little use. At one point when she needed to go to the bathroom she simply tried to stand to walk and fell, failing to realize what was wrong.

When a doctor misinterpreted her garbled speech during rounds one day Paula thought he turned to a nurse saying, "Paula can't understand you and probably never will." She was furious, wanting somehow to communicate this was not so, with anger turning to frustration when no words came to express her feelings. Now, she wonders if she could have misinterpreted his words because of her poor comprehension abilities.

Paula's parents and family coped as best they could during the three months she stayed in the rehabilitation unit. Since the hospital was some distance away from their home, much time was spent driving back and forth daily. The family was under continuing stress with her parents away from home and two children still living there. As Paula began to get better, though, she began to recognize family members, easing some of the alienation from her they had felt for so long. Finally, in December, 1982, Paula was discharged and returned home—four months after surgery.

Tom

It took two weeks after Tom Martin collapsed at home and was rushed to the hospital for him to recognize anyone in his family. The crisis started one night in August, 1983, when Tom had a headache so severe that "I was up all night taking drugs and hot showers trying to get some relief." Nothing seemed to help, and the next morning as he was getting ready for work, he collapsed in the tub. His son heard the fall and rushed to the bathroom. By that time Tom couldn't move his right side and was rapidly losing his speech. Tommy summoned a neighbor and they drove him to the hospital, frightened and bewildered. Although medical tests confirmed a stroke in the left temporal parietal area of his brain, the exact cause was not determined. Except for a history of heavy cigarette smoking, Tom had always been active and enjoyed excellent health.

Tom's family stayed in his hospital room around the clock, looking each day for any hopeful sign that he was responding. The first sign Lee saw came with a present from him, sent through her mother-in-law. Somehow Tom had communicated that he wanted to give his wife a wooden duck to add to her collection. Lee knew then that "he was going to make it. He was still thinking, he simply had no language, so he needed to show me in other ways." Days later they celebrated a friend's birthday in Tom's room, and his first words came when he sang "Happy Birthday" with the others. (This stimulation is used frequently by speech and language pathologists who hope to get someone to use words again. Hearing a well-learned tune accesses the unaffected right hemisphere of the brain responsible for melody, and recall of the tune can automatically trigger expression of the corresponding words.)

As Tom began to respond more, he was supported by visiting friends. Lee was uncertain how to react to this outpouring of love from others. "I am a private person. I seem to handle crisis by withdrawing into myself . . . I appreciated the support, but didn't know how to handle the steady stream of visitors." As she looks back on this time, she realizes "how much I was retreating from everyone." She feels this may have been misinterpreted by some as a desire that they not visit. As time went on and she began to relax more, she watched these friends drift away, perhaps because she seemed to close them out during those early weeks. This can happen easily; friends wish to offer support but are unsure what is appropriate. Since the family is immersed in the crisis and may not know or say what they need, it is best that friends respond the way *they* feel most comfortable, aware that, like Lee, family members may not react the way they think and/or wish they would.

Tom gradually came to understand the gravity of his condition; as a pharmacist he knew about strokes and aphasia. He seemed unable to control his outpouring of emotion. Furthermore, his thinking was so "foggy" that he assumed he was saying what he was thinking, and when he spoke he was puzzled by the lack of response from others. When people spoke to him he was not able to differentiate words, yet he noticed the tone of their voices and appreciated that he was included. He also came to realize his right side was paralyzed and spastic; the spasticity made his limbs resist bending—they could only extend. The severity of his stroke warranted intensive rehabilitation, but this necessary treatment was difficult for him at first since he was still too sick, fatigued, and oblivious to his surroundings to understand the extent of his limitations.

Tom spent eight weeks on various medical floors where he felt "isolated without any connection to the hospital staff." He sensed that the staff treated him as "something less than human," and he felt like crying out: "I am a human being, too!" Tom's sense of the reactions of the staff may have been exaggerated, for during his illness and hospitalization, he felt so "out of control" about every aspect of his life that he may have projected his own feelings about himself onto the staff. Thus Tom really did feel "less than human" as he lay helpless in his bed and sensed that those caring for him were responding likewise. The demands on hospital personnel can be so intense that often more of their time may be spent with those patients who interact with them more easily. It would be impossible to determine what actually occurred, but Tom does recall one speech and language pathologist who seemed to understand and treat him as an "equal." The sensitivity of that staff member did much to motivate his recovery.

Tom was next moved to the rehabilitation unit, where he stayed for six weeks. By this time he was more motivated to get better and remembers his daughter's constant presence and support. Since Lee was now back at work, the help of friends and family members was essential to the Martins. Tom recalls having to "sit around and wait for therapies," but most other memories of this time are vague. Tom returned home in November, 1983, three and a half months after his stroke, unable to speak and understand what others were saying and still confined to a wheelchair.

Carl

On August 2, 1984, Carl Wilson had successful heart by-pass surgery. Earlier his doctor had diagnosed major blockage in an artery leading to the heart and had recommended the operation as a means to reduce a substantial risk of heart attack. As usual, Carl viewed this choice as a matter of fact decision, wanting to "get his plumbing fixed" so he could get on with life. He was more concerned with the day after surgery, not the procedure itself, fearful of developing pneumonia.

It was no surprise to his brother that Carl had packed brief-cases full of work when he called him into his office the night before admission to the hospital. Carl explained the simplicity of the procedure and the small risk of complication. He told his brother, who worked for him, to continue on as best he could with the company should anything happen. Later at home his wife and daughters found themselves reassured and supported by a husband and father who was composed as usual.

Early on August 4, though, as Carl was sitting in a chair in his hospital room brushing his teeth, he became weak and confused. He did not abruptly lose consciousness—rather, as in many stroke cases, lethargy increased gradually as time passed. His daughter, Kristen, remembers being awakened at home by her mother with the news that her father was not doing well. She suddenly found herself too afraid to ask about his condition but on the way to the hospital painfully watched her mother's tears as the word "stroke" was said for the first time. When they walked into the hospital room Carl's eyes were open, seemingly filled with fear. He was able to squeeze their hands but his right arm wandered with uncontrolled movement. As physicians gathered by Carl's bed, Kristen, concerned that they were "talking over" her father, asked them to include him in the conversation. At this point she wanted to deny this was happening—he was her daddy and he *had* to understand. The family watched in horror while Carl drifted further away each hour.

Carl himself has no memory of this. It has been helpful in his emotional recovery to hear his family recount these moments many times, giving reassurance that it is normal for him to have no memories of the time and that it is unlikely that he will ever suddenly remember it.

Eileen remembers the shock and denial of this period. She found herself feeling her life had ended as her total emotional dependency on Carl was abruptly severed. She was convinced she simply couldn't go on without Carl telling her how to live her life and solving her problems. She learned her husband had a "massive" stroke but what did this mean—would he live?

Kristen, the oldest daughter, found herself caught in the conflict of two roles. As a registered nurse, she was aware that the IV bottles, settings on the ventilator, and the presence of other equipment indicated someone who was seriously ill. She felt she needed to be strong—ask the appropriate questions, get the clinical facts, and support her mother, who was barely standing at this point. Yet when the neurologist told them the diagnosis was "massive stroke," her own feelings were too strong to hold back. Not knowing what else to do, she closed herself in a phone booth to cry. As her emotions came it was too hard to make the medical care seem routine and positive for everyone. The situation was now personal.

Eventually doctors found the cause of Carl's stroke: an embolus had blocked one branch of his left carotid artery, disrupting the blood supply to the entire left hemisphere of the brain. Carl lost consciousness for seven days, requiring respirator support. When he regained consciousness, he had a "global" aphasia, meaning he could not produce any speech or writing, recognize any written words, and had only a minimal understanding of what others were saying to him. The right side of his body was paralyzed as well.

As the days of hospitalization drifted into weeks, each family member experienced different reactions. Eileen gradually realized she had to start making decisions she never thought she could. She found the avenue of direct confrontation best, letting herself risk making "wrong" decisions. She knew it was important and necessary to "just keep making them."

Kristen recalls the need to blame. Since her father had had surgery prior to the stroke it was easy to think about blaming the surgeon, nurses, anyone in the hospital. She even blamed her father for having the surgery. Laying blame is a normal part of grief as people begin to deal with loss following a major crisis. It was also crucial to her that hospital staff get an idea of the man behind the equipment, so she brought pictures of her father to tape to the walls in the hope the nurses could gain an understanding of Carl's personality. She was facing the loss of her father's control by attempting to bring some of the normal outside world into this sterile hospital setting.

Daughter Susan's strongest reaction to the stroke was that someone was missing. "It was as if Dad was away on a trip and would be coming back and the person in intensive care was not anyone I knew." Families of stroke survivors frequently describe a depersonalization effect that occurs in response to seeing a loved one gravely ill. Life-support equipment, bodily tone and postural changes with paralysis, and loss of the ability to communicate can all result in a person who no longer looks or sounds the same. The family struggles as it begins to come to terms with the sudden loss of a known personality.

Carl's brother, Allen, found medical language incomprehensible, yet he yearned for information in order to understand, cope, and renew hope. He feels the family would have been more confused and upset if Kristen hadn't been able to translate terminology for them. Susan was confused by the care of several different physicians—neurologist, surgeon, internist—expressing a need to feel that "someone was in charge of Dad's case overall." She felt much appreciation for the medical care the nurses were offering but wanted someone to help her understand what was going on with her father's body and address her continual fears that he would become worse and die. At times she wished the nurses "knew what it felt like to have someone they loved in a situation like this."

Graduation to a private room, sitting in a wheelchair, or going outside for the first time became momentous things. Holding playing cards, moving the wheelchair, and taking off a shirt were no longer acts just taken for granted. Like most stroke survivors, Carl needed much encouragement to redevelop and celebrate accomplishment of these seemingly trivial skills. It was easy for him to be engrossed only in the present, as much energy had to be directed toward movements and thoughts that were previously automatic. For this reason stroke survivors often lose perspective as to how much progress has actually been made. Reminders from others can be invaluable.

Susan was confused over when to give feedback about progress and how honest she should be. Although she was elated when he was able to get into a wheelchair for the first time she was hesitant to show her happiness, fearing her dad saw it as a reminder of his current limitations. She also struggled with the notion that he might be having different thoughts, or that he felt bothered by so much attention from family. As do most family members, Susan had to cope not only with the illness but also with her own emotional reactions to it.

Eileen first felt this conflict when she gave her husband a comb. He immediately put it under his nose instead of in his hair and she was reminded of an old joke between them when he used to do an imitation. Eileen laughed, then tried to stop, mortified because she felt, "I'm not supposed to laugh." She was no longer sure if Carl was repeating the old joke or if he was actually having trouble using the comb correctly. There was nothing wrong with Eileen's laughter, but she was uncertain if it should be expressed. It might have helped her to talk about this with the rest of her family. Sharing emotional reactions to this illness helps family members draw together, give one another suggestions, and remind each that he is not alone in his uncertainty and fear.

After one month Carl was transferred to the rehabilitation unit. His personality was beginning to blossom again, leading to his constant push to improve. In the unit the emphasis turned to effort and accomplishment. Carl's brother learned to think, "one day at a time," and to notice the small changes each day brought. He had difficulty withdrawing his help at times to let Carl try doing for himself; it was painful to watch someone he loved go through laboriously slow struggles. Carl, however, quickly reestablished some degree of independence and control by making it clear when he wanted to attempt something on his own.

His family learned how to help with exercises during their visits. Since stroke survivors need frequent short periods of stimulation, the more family or friends can supplement formal therapy sessions the better. Not everyone responds well to this, however. For some, the emotional reactions in working with a close loved one are too great, causing additional stress. In such a case it may be better for another person to help with exercises, but Carl took to working with family well. He began to request that his daughters do exercises with him.

Kristen remembers her dismay as her father was placed back on a monitor following a brief period of unresponsiveness in the wheelchair one day. Her strength, coming from the knowledge that he was getting better, quickly drained. It was very tough for her to once again entertain doubts. As time passed Carl went through many of these fluctuations. One day he was in good spirits and the next felt frustrated: sometimes able to laugh, sometimes depressed. His daughter learned these fluctuations were an expected part of recovery and did not mean regression.

Susan remembers that as time passed burnout occurred within the family. This is common because of the continuous energy needed over an extended period of time. As her family attempted to work together, she saw them "get on each other's nerves" more quickly. Life began to feel like a series of tragedies, and the long hours seemed too hard. Carl had always told her she could come to him whatever the problem and now her source of strength seemed gone. She eventually found strength through the family bond and by thinking of reversed roles with her father; he had given of himself to raise her; now she needed to do the same for him.

Relearning activities of daily living was stressed in the rehabilitation unit in preparation for discharge. Dressing, feeding, grooming, moving the wheelchair, transferring to a chair, standing, communicating, and the beginnings of social interaction with other patients and staff were part of the daily routine. Eileen and Kristen were thrilled the first time Carl stood up. Therapists helped them prepare for the possibility of a fall by having them help Carl up from the floor.

Eileen remembers her elation when Carl was able to begin coming home for weekend visits. But, as the other stroke survivors and their families found, this was also terrifying. She just didn't feel she had enough knowledge and skill to deal with Carl at home even though the weekend visits served as a transition to hospital discharge. Family education sessions were held with nurses, therapists, and the physician; in fact, a final family conference before discharge was scheduled. Carl's daughter remembers how nervous they were about meeting with all health professionals at once and about the information they would be told. She remembers this as one of the toughest and most disheartening days of the entire experience. As a family they had prepared a list of questions, but when the meeting started they felt barraged with information about Carl's limitations. They were told he would spend the rest of his life in a wheelchair and would never have speech again. When the meeting ended they left for home feeling drained. Susan felt some positive messages or encouragement would have helped her family to keep motivated. Instead, it took them some time to rebuild strength to continue coping with Carl's illness after he at last returned home.

Conclusion

Sharing these families' memories in the early, acute stages of this illness, it is clear that many of their emotional reactions and concerns are universal. For nearly all, this was the first time they had seen a stroke. The sudden onset and seriousness of it proved frightening, contributing to their confusion. Since these first memories associated with abrupt change and crisis are permanent, it is important for the well-being of everyone that others respond with patience and understanding.

They all needed to feel a human connection between themselves and hospital personnel. For the aphasic person, who no longer understands spoken language, nonverbal communication becomes more important. Eye contact, tone of voice, touching, taking time to just "be with" them (as the nurse's aide did for Betty that lonely night) can form a bridge to make an important human connection.

Our families also expressed a desire to be informed as early as possible about the medical diagnosis, preferably in a quiet, private place, with an explanation of the medical condition in familiar terms. This contact contributed to their feelings of worth and helped establish them as integral parts in the recovery. Most patients and families preferred to hear both good and bad news in a direct manner along with words of encouragement. They felt this communication was important to nurture motivation and strength in themselves and the stroke survivor.

During hospitalization and subsequent rehabilitation, as in these cases, several health care professionals may interact with the stroke survivor and family. Medical doctors who may see a person after a stroke include physiatrists, internists, neurologists, and neurosurgeons. Physiatrists are specialists in physical medicine and rehabilitation; they examine those stroke survivors with weakness or paralysis and often will then prescribe physical and/or occupational therapy. An internist is a doctor who specializes in internal medicine and will, in most cases, oversee the total health care of his patients. In addition, consultation with neurologists, who diagnose and treat diseases of the brain, and with neurosurgeons, who perform brain surgery, may be part of medical rehabilitation.

Stroke survivors will see other health care professionals in addition to their physicians. A speech and language pathologist will consult when aphasia is present and will diagnose and treat deficits in all areas of communication. Occupational therapists and physical therapists treat patients with paralysis and hemiparesis. (In cases of stroke with aphasia this will most often affect the right side.) An occupational therapist addresses physical and visual perceptual deficits that affect the return of functional skills needed daily. He works to restore strength and mobility and to teach the utilization of compensatory devices that will aid the return of such skills as self-care, the performance of household chores, and driving. A physical therapist treats the return of the functioning of the arm and leg, checking and working with a stroke survivor's balance in all positions. His role is to help maintain flexibility, strengthen muscles, and specifically teach patients how to minimize tone loss in the affected muscles. Other rehabilitation professionals that may be part of the staff are music, art, and recreational therapists, each of whom functions to restore mental and physical health to the stroke survivor.

Patients and families are experiencing loss, grief, and sadness while they are trying to learn an overwhelming amount of new information to cope with their situation. Health care professionals cannot solve all the problems associated with the illness, nor should patients and families be forced to respond to accommodate the needs of the hospital. The hospital staff should be available to accompany them on their journey, providing information and support as needed. There may be a broad range of individual responses—from disbelief and denial to rage and anger—and it is important that patients and families feel comfortable expressing all emotions. What may appear to be excessive denial of the present condition may, in reality, be a needed defense to protect against information too overwhelming to hear at this stage of recovery. Each emotional reaction needs to be recognized and fully experienced. Time will lessen the intensity of these initial feelings.

Because this is a highly emotional time for everyone, misunderstandings between staff and families can and do occur. Often information needs to be repeated more than once. In addition, the aphasic individual may not understand or retain what he hears. It is important to remember that the person with aphasia *can* understand the *intent* of the message and should therefore be included in family conferences even at this early stage. Providing written information helps reduce misunderstandings.

In fact, these families found writing about these events while in the hospital to be helpful, and many kept a journal. This record of events and feelings can help to organize internally what is often a chaotic time. Questions and concerns can be written down so they are ready when staff is available. Since memory is often taxed under stress, this journal can serve as a backup. Finally, the journal can later be shared with the stroke survivor, reviewing events he may have little recollection or understanding of during his hospital stay.

3.

Homecoming

Although the time in the hospital varied for each person, the average length of stay for Paula, Ed, Tom, Carl, Ted, and Betty was three months. Three months full of changes. For each of them, it was a period to heal from the acute stage of his illness. For their families, it was a period of adjustment to a new way of living. Most of the families remember a continuous struggle in attempting to balance a life at home with one at the hospital. While there were opportunities during their hospital stay for weekend day and/or night passes home, most stroke survivors felt that after the brief visit it was comforting to know they had some place to return. This once "foreign territory" had become a "home" of sorts, or at least a place to feel nurtured and secure during the first phase of recovery. Therefore, when it was finally time to go home for good, this separation from the hospital was viewed with some trepidation by both the stroke survivors and their families.

This much-anticipated event, while a sign of improvement, is still another change to face. A stroke survivor may feel frightened about leaving a sheltered environment, for though he is better, he is different than he was before the illness. Dr. Oliver Sacks (1984), a neurologist and the author of *A Leg to Stand On*, who was hospitalized in a rehabilitation facility for an extended period, describes his own fears about leaving the hospital: "All of us were 'eager to leave', eager to get out, and get on to the next step. And yet this involved a relinquishing of the care, of the cherished infant status we were now used to. We wanted, consciously, to be weaned, but unconsciously we feared, and tried to stop it, to prolong our special pampered status."

According to our families, even those who received the best of care and were well prepared for discharge, information about living with this disability was incomplete. It was difficult for them to anticipate their own needs at a time when they were too overwhelmed to assimilate everything required by the new situation. Many felt abruptly cut off from the specialized care received in the hospital, for not only were their main supports gone but the new faces and new routines of outpatient rehabilitation had now to be reckoned with.

Dr. Sacks reveals more of his feelings about hospital discharge in the following:

> It was not enough to be physically well, if we still felt the fear and the cares of the ill. We had all, in our ways, been undermined by sickness—had lost all the careless boldness, the freedom, of the well . . . We had to have an in between, a place where we could live a limited but steadily enlarging existence—until we were ready to reenter the great world . . . We needed a quiet place, a haven, a shelter where we could gradually regain our confidence and our health, our confidence no less than our health.

Our families' own experiences in coping with the first few months at home are enlightening. Many experienced this loss of self-confidence described so well by Dr. Sacks. Most expressed fears and concerns about returning to the familiarity of home, a place comforting yet foreign since they themselves were now so changed. Once home, each room flashed memories of a self that had once moved about with relative ease. These memories created fears and doubts about the future—questions and concerns that were to last several months. What physical changes needed to be made in the house? How should friends and extended family become acquainted with this disabling illness? How would changes in day-to-day living be faced? What additional problems might arise? In the following chapter each of our families shares the solutions that helped make the transition smoother.

Physical Preparations

As the time to return home approached, some families first had to make changes at home. Carl, Tom and Paula's homes needed alterations so they could move about in their wheelchairs. Paula's downstairs living room was made into a bedroom for the first year. Her family had to order a hospital bed and other medical supplies, such as a commode chair. Since she had been ill for so long prior to the brain surgery and had needed special considerations at that time also, these adjustments were not big ones for her family.

It was more of an emotional struggle for Carl's wife to adapt when the master bedroom was moved to the first-floor dining room and their dining room furniture moved upstairs. So much of her life had already shifted, she reacted to the changes in her home as a great loss. Some feel perplexed when emotional reactions seem disproportionate to the event; remembering that we become protective of *any* stability we still have following change helps.

In Tom's case everyone desperately tried to make things as "normal" as possible even though they obviously weren't. The day he left the hospital with his family his daughter remembers: "We all cried all the way home." After struggling to transfer from the car to his wheelchair, Tom thought the three steps to their front door suddenly seemed larger and steeper than before. Although his family was advised to build a ramp to accommodate the wheelchair, Tom hadn't wanted this, thinking it would only remind him of his disability. Instead, Lee somehow lifted him— wheelchair and all—up those stairs the first day and every day until he was able to walk them himself. Looking back, she has no idea how she managed, since her husband weighs over two hundred pounds! Eventually Tom was able to descend those steps, first by sitting down and then by walking with the support of a railing.

A second adaptation was the installation of a shower chair to make bathing easier. After Tom was helped into the bathtub, he could sit alone on this chair while he bathed, leaving his family free from worry that he might fall. For the first month a home health aide tended to Tom's personal care, but he soon learned from his occupational therapist to take over his own dressing, bathing, and grooming. (Home health aides, who can provide a useful resource for care during the transition to home life, are available in most communities and may be covered by health insurance. This service can ease burdens in an already emotionally and physically taxed family. Adult day care might be another option for those who have no one to help with care during the day. Although none of our families used these services, Tom's family might have needed them if his mother had not been available after Lee's return to work.)

Early Memories

Those stroke survivors who were more aware of the extent of their illness were better prepared both for what they faced coming home and for outpatient rehabilitation. Those still too ill often remember nothing until the brain has had more time to heal.

Paula remembers nothing of the day she left the hospital but finds her first memories in driving home from a doctor's appointment with her father. As they pulled into the driveway, she watched the delivery of the commode chair, knowing there was something peculiar about this strange piece of furniture but finding it impossible to make any sense out of what she saw. Carl doesn't remember the day of his homecoming and his recollections of the first few months are unclear. He knows he slept a lot, and that his early routine consisted of learning to transfer from bed to wheelchair only to return to bed once again.

As Ed and Julie drove home from the hospital, Ed's first memory was of seeing his mailbox with *his* address on *his* house. "It felt great!" Julie laughed away his first remark, that she was going to have to "tell me what everything in the house is because I don't know," until later, when watching him wander through each room, she realized just how little recognition he actually had of the things in their house or the names of them.

Ted's homecoming is his first clear memory. He was devastated by how he looked and felt "completely disconnected from everyone and everything." He also recalls just wanting to sleep and a heady sensation that he was "flying all the time." He wasn't interested in T.V. because there was no understanding of what he heard and he was so easily distracted. Alice watched him as he drifted aimlessly though their house: "I just didn't know what to do with him!" In this situation it was an understandable reaction for Alice to want Ted "to do something!" to make her feel better, because activity seemed more "normal." But at this time Ted was far from normal and really needed relief from the constant barrage of auditory and visual stimulation that is part of everyone's life. His family had trouble realizing just how confusing and overwhelming it was to face the "real world" once again. Ted needed time to try to make sense out of a life that was familiar, yet one he was now seeing from a new perspective.

Ted also felt like "everyone was always watching me!" He had limited awareness that he was bumping into everything because of the reduced visual field on his right side. He also kept missing the steps on the front porch and occasionally landed on the cement or fell while going up the stairs to his bedroom. This made his family even more nervous, causing them to watch him more closely to prevent any injuries. Ted was also "cold all the time," no matter how high the heat was turned on in the house. Many say they experience this change in thermal regulation but notice that this sensation seems to go away over time. Those with a hemiparesis appear to have more of a continuing problem regulating body temperature.

Betty's fondest memory was of sleeping in her own bed again—the worst was of planning and preparing meals. Since her husband had had serious medical problems for some time before her stroke, he seemed even more helpless and forgetful with this new trauma. With her support of him now taken away he was not able to help, and Betty needed to assist him in buying and preparing their meals. While Bill was able to drive her to the store, Betty was often not able to make it down all the aisles. She'd load up on prepared meals and arrive home sometimes with an odd assortment of foods. In addition, she was bewildered at times over how to manage cooking with one arm: "All I knew was that I had no choice but to learn and to learn *fast.*" Her occupational therapist taught her to use a cutting board adapted for one hand, which helped her to slice. (Tom also got this kind of help and uses a knife with a curved blade for cutting his meat and another adaptive device to help him open jars.) Other devices were also available for use in the kitchen. Betty checked local stores carrying these aids and asked her occupational therapist how to use them most effectively. Betty can laugh now when she looks back on earlier experiments: "And I don't think I can ever look at another T.V. dinner again!" But nothing was funny at the time about her struggles, struggles that ended in exhaustion and many nights overwhelmed her.

First Emotional Reactions

A wide range of emotional responses was connected with the return home. Some reactions were expected while others were a surprise.

In Ed's house the physical surroundings stayed the same since he had very little remaining weakness on his right side. Things were the same—and yet somehow they weren't. Ed had more visual problems than many stroke survivors and with his visual field reduced on his right side, he had to remember to turn his head in order to take in all his surroundings. Often he forgot and missed objects he was searching for. He found simple actions like looking at a clock difficult, for first he had trouble locating it and then couldn't recognize the time when he did. In addition, he had trouble accurately perceiving what he saw. Julie remembers one incident shortly after his homecoming. As Ed was dressing he saw his toe poking through a hole in his sock but could make no sense of it. Incredulous, he asked Julie, "What happened to my doorknob?" She began to laugh, then saw that her husband was hurt by her laughter. Realizing his sensitivity and the terrible sense of confusion he must be feeling, she asked, "Ed, it's either laugh or cry; which do you want?" He, in turn, broke into laughter. Julie feels they rediscovered the healing value of laughter that day. From then on, as they shared his recovery, they also shared their laughter: "laugh and let it go!"

In Carl's household, Eileen was struggling to regain hope and motivation after "the worst day of my life." The family conference in the rehabilitation unit that day before discharge had sent her spirits lower than ever. "You could have scraped me off the floor . . . I wish they had been more compassionate . . . , even given us false hope instead of no hope . . . then further down the road I could have dealt with it." Already apprehensive about Carl's homecoming, Eileen felt the content and timing of this final meeting only served to increase her stress. As he came home just before the Christmas holidays, she kept thinking about how this holiday would be so different from last year's. Although she had been inundated with information from the medical staff, she really had no idea how she was going to deal with this "new" person at home. In fact, the first two to three months were filled with seesawing emotions—the thrill of having her husband home alternating with fear for his well-being and doubt of her own capability to handle him. She describes this time as one of the most difficult for her. She worried constantly about things that might go wrong and was frightened about what she would do if he fell. When this happened for the first time, they were both able to handle it, having had the opportunity to practice getting up off the floor in physical therapy. Her fear of Carl hurting himself was understandable after dealing with the necessary period of dependency and caretaking following the stroke. It was a natural instinct to protect, even overprotect, against the possibility of further loss and pain. What needs to be recognized is that most persons *do* have the coping skills necessary to deal with all these changes, as Eileen was surprised to learn.

Another unexpected emotional response for Eileen was her utter confusion as to how to handle her husband's anger. When it started she was completely unprepared, never having seen Carl have "temper tantrums." As his shouting and pounding on the table escalated, Eileen tried to calm him, but nothing worked. This was before she learned that most stroke survivors go through periods of anger during recovery. Because Carl was still so ill, he does not remember these episodes, and when his family gathered to talk about this book, they shared their memories with him. It was very hard for him to hear what he had put his family through, but it helped in all their healing to review these memories. All had to remember that his anger was not directed at them personally; rather, it was a generalized reaction to the loss that Carl had experienced, and any attempts to suppress it were of little help. There was really nothing Eileen could do except "wait it out." Many find it helps to let the family member know how upsetting this expression of anger is to them. The stroke survivor may not stop, but at least the family's difficulties in dealing with this behavior have been honestly communicated. This is a time when families need to find support from others in order to talk about frustrations and release them.

As for her own emotional expression, Eileen worked hard to constantly appear "up" to Carl. She cried a lot, but only by herself. Although it was a strain on her, Eileen believed she should not show her own anger, sadness, or frustration. Now she expresses these emotions freely. Early on, she believes it would have helped to know that such expression of real feelings does not interfere with recovery. On the contrary, a return to real human interaction aids the stroke survivor in expressing his own real feelings and helps to reestablish familiar patterns of relating to one another. There are so many conflicting emotions during this period of recovery that suppression of emotions will not help the healing.

Carl and Eileen's children remember well the adjustments they made when their father came home. Marsha felt happy but uncomfortable at the same time. She saw her father, formerly a symbol of authority, now totally dependent on others. She found her own strength to face this misfortune developing over time (she had met her husband the same year and found added support in this new relationship) but missed and still misses the sense of direction, leadership, and presence of her father. It was also painful for her to watch her parents dissolve the family business and have to sell the home and farm. She still resents what she felt to be "point-blank negative assessment" from the medical staff at discharge, but she felt inspired by her father's courage. She has now seen him surpass all medical predictions and feels his personal strength was the driving force that got him where he is today.

One of Susan's reactions to her father's homecoming was fear for her mother—she was unsure how Eileen would physically and emotionally care for him day after day. This daily care also took so long that there was no time left for simply enjoying each other's company as before. Time helped her develop trust when she saw Eileen taking care of herself, too.

As Carl improved, his awareness increased. He *hated* the need "to be taken care of." While it was difficult for him to give up his independence, it was also important for him to remain well-groomed. To this day, Carl expresses appreciation to his home health aides for helping him to retain his dignity by "looking good" when he was so disabled. Often the family is so engrossed in meeting physical needs that they forget how important grooming can be to someone who is ill. Paying attention to this important detail is time well spent toward increasing feelings of self-worth.

The Lamberts all remember Ted's homecoming as a time of emotional turmoil. Since Sid hated his father's sudden temper outbursts, which occurred when Ted was trying to make his family understand something, he avoided home at first. His brother Allen wanted to avoid sitting at the dinner table with his dad because it was simply too painful to watch how sloppily he ate and that he forgot to finish the food on the right side of his plate. Allen was also nervous about having his dad home, feeling that the medical staff knew more about this and that he wouldn't know what to do if something happened.

Sometimes a stroke survivor can feel so devastated by his current condition that he is unaware of the demands he places on others. This happened to Tom, who remembers how difficult it was moving in the cramped quarters of his house in a wheelchair. Since he felt so physically restricted, he began ordering the family to get him things and got angry when they didn't come immediately. While it might have helped for his family members to explain their perspective, they probably would have had to reiterate their feelings several times before Tom would have remembered. As Tom recovered he slowly became more aware that other family members had their own needs.

Tom's daughter, Stacey, found the first months to be the most difficult. While she had seen her dad daily in the hospital, she could leave whenever she became too emotionally and physically drained—now "he was always there." She felt estranged from her school friends, who couldn't really understand her father's stroke, and found herself more and more alone.

In Tom's case feelings of alienation were overwhelming when he attempted to reintegrate himself into the family routines because he sensed that they were "okay . . . without me." He was no longer included in the family's planning and decision-making because of his limited communication, and their busy schedules often didn't allow time for them to give lengthy explanations to Tom. He pounded the arms of a living room chair one day in utter frustration, not knowing how else to cope with his feelings.

Betty was emotionally drained during those first months. Realizing the extent of her husband's deteriorating physical and mental health was difficult enough, but during that time her sister, who had been her main support through her illness, was diagnosed with and died of cancer. Later that same year, her brother also died. Looking at her other losses, "I just didn't seem to have the emotional reserves left to cope with death." Unfortunately, as Betty was learning, "one serious trauma does not insulate you from others." Somehow she survived this time, with her husband's children playing a significant role. Because Betty was always so self-sufficient, she really didn't know how to ask for their help, and she will long remember that they were there to give their support. Important learning came at this time when she became able to reach out to others and receive what they offered.

Some of the stroke survivors entertained thoughts of suicide. Ted and Tom both thought about taking their own lives during that first year. They felt useless in not being able to care for their families as before. When Ted developed another illness (unrelated to the stroke) that required hospitalization, the pain reliever he was given appeared to aggravate his depression, and he warned his wife when he returned home to throw away all medicine in the house. At that point, he didn't trust himself to be alone in his sadness. Tom's son, who was at first responsible for driving him, heard threats on several occasions that his dad was going to jump out of the car. He was frightened and not sure what his father was capable of doing. Sometimes suicidal thoughts need to be addressed by a professional as the stroke survivor works through his grief; those working with him should be made aware of any expression of these suicidal feelings so that an appropriate referral can be made if needed. (Chapter 5, "Psychosocial Issues Related to Stroke and Aphasia," contains more information about counseling.)

Changing Relationships

Most of the stroke survivors talked about changes in their relationships with other family members. In Ed's case, those who were not able to accept his illness withdrew from him, but he and Julie hope these relationships will change with time. Some family members responded by taking extra time to invite him over or call him on the phone. Ed felt the special love of his grandchildren, especially in the first few months after the stroke, when their unconditional love helped motivate him through this sad and difficult time. He recalls with amusement the reaction of one grandson when he found out that "Grandpa could not read." The child climbed on his lap with *The Three Little Pigs* and read it to him, assuring Grandpa that he would teach him how to read again. Children who have not yet learned to inhibit their response to serious illness and disability can play a special role in recovery, often expressing through their curiosity what other family members and friends are afraid to say.

After her return home, Paula found her family had "to learn more about aphasia in order to communicate with me." It was discouraging to her family to realize how little she actually understood. Cathy, her younger sister, felt guilty when she became irritated over Paula's constant agreement with everything she said. When they realized the severity of her auditory comprehension problem, they finally understood that communication was going to be a hit-or-miss affair. During the roughest times it was hard to reconcile conflicting feelings. In the Sams's family, as in other families who experience the devastation of a stroke, individual needs as well as the needs of the family cannot always be met. Pain and withdrawal occurred in spite of the best intentions of everyone. Paula's niece, to whom she had been very close before the stroke, was frightened by all the hospital equipment and would not visit. Her brother John knew Paula needed everyone's support, but missed the company of his parents, who were now too busy to spend time with him and his family. Holidays were particularly difficult when his parent had to leave after a couple of hours to take Paula home to bed. He resented that she would not rest at his house to avoid breaking up the family gathering.

Cathy, too, felt conflicting emotions about her sister's illness. Before this happened, Paula had been a "second mother" to her since their own mother had been recovering from brain surgery herself for several years. Now, as a young teenager, she watched the nightmare of serious illness disrupt the family again; her "second" mother too was disabled. Cathy was supportive at first but eventually felt overwhelmed by the situation; she found herself caught in a web of emotions she didn't fully understand and ultimately withdrew from the family. Alone and disillusioned, she attempted to take her own life. Paula's mother is still saddened over realization of just how alone Cathy felt. "Her illness, unlike Paula's, was inside, it couldn't be seen . . . , and I didn't know she needed our help. We didn't know what to do." Cathy thinks her conflict may have stemmed from guilt she felt over her anger about the family's past situation. She loved Paula and wanted to help her, but at times found herself resenting her for becoming ill and needing so much attention.

Tom's mother often drove her son to therapy sessions and remembers her pain as she watched him struggling to recover. "It should have been me, not my son. I was afraid to ask questions, afraid that I really didn't want to know how bad it was." The less she knew, the less she would have to deal with. Because of her sorrow, she wanted to overprotect him. This created conflict with her daughter-in-law, who had to return to work full-time and needed Tom to be more independent. Eventually, Lee helped her see that Tom needed to do things for himself in order to increase his self-respect.

Fatigue after Stroke

Fatigue seemed to be an issue for everyone because the stroke survivors still needed extra rest and their concerned families at times interpreted extra sleeping as emotional withdrawal. Tom and Betty both talked about this fatigue as a feeling beyond "just needing sleep." More often than not, it was a sudden loss of ability to function at all. It would come without warning, so intense and alarming that they felt like retreating from everyone and everything.

The spouse or the major caregiver, on the other hand, can become exhausted from the added responsibilities and the effects of emotional stress. In Julie's case, even though additional rest would have helped, she just couldn't find the time to fit it into her busy schedule. A substitute to resting may include finding time alone, perhaps asking a friend or another family member to take over responsibility for "caring" for awhile. While many feel guilty leaving, going out even for a brief time breaks the routine and offers a chance to see things from a new perspective. Julie found she returned with more energy to put into the relationship after leaving to enjoy herself for a few hours.

Ed slept often at first and even now continues to take naps two to three times a day. Paula found herself continually struggling through fatigue to get "everything I had to do done." Although she always reminded herself that she was "going to achieve whatever goal I set for myself," she constantly had to remember to allow more time. After two years this was somewhat better; after four years she was able to "go all day and crash at bedtime." Now, "I get up at 7:00 and go through the whole day." She has learned to pace herself, since too many busy days in a row will bring on exhaustion. Having learned to listen to her body when she is out, she will first sit down to rest when tired, then excuse herself to go home early. Although she would still like to have greater endurance, social functions don't have to be avoided this way—she can enjoy herself for the period of time her body will tolerate.

Lee noted that while Tom continued to get fatigued, when their life together eased from its initial frantic pace after the stroke, she was less tired with a resumed interest in becoming more involved socially. Since the pace of their lives now differed, she and Tom found it helpful to discuss this difference. Arrangements could then be made beforehand for her to attend a social function alone or for Tom to go too for a shorter time. If this issue is addressed early, open communication should result in less tension.

In Tom's case, though his fatigue remains almost constant, he "keeps going!" At times when "I simply can't do another thing," he reminds himself that "pushing to the limit" is partially responsible for his dramatic recovery. During the first couple of years, his family was particularly frustrated by Tom's refusal to admit he was tired. Fixated on an idea, he would not let it go even as he watched the frustration and despair of his family while they attempted to reason with him. In this case, Tom was too tired even to recognize his own confusion. Now he works toward becoming more aware of his fatigue so that he can postpone important discussions or decisions until he can fully concentrate.

Establishing Routines

Each of us has routines that make our day-to-day existence run smoothly and allow us to deal more effectively with unexpected events. But our families' normal routines were disrupted following the stroke. Most would have felt more comfortable if they could have reestablished their familiar patterns once their family member returned home, but this was not always possible. As they strove to regain some degree of normalcy, they sought ways of reestablishing routines that would help them gain strength to continue coping with the crisis.

Eileen, for example, had long anticipated her first good night's sleep in months once Carl was home. Instead, sleeping became far more difficult. Carl's hemiparesis made sleeping in their habitual positions impossible and limited his ability to move. Eileen awoke several times each night, fearful that her husband might have a problem, checking to make sure he was still breathing—much as she had done with her babies years before.

Spouses often have difficulty sleeping through the night. Many times they must assist their spouse to the bathroom or help him use a urinal or bedpan. Since adequate sleep is important for the major caregiver, who must continue to think clearly and function with his added responsibilities, he may have to consider alternatives to preserve his emotional and physical health. Hiring someone to help at night or having the stroke survivor take care of his own bedpan or urinal when he is able might be options. At this early stage in his recovery, the stroke survivor can be unaware of the extra time required from the spouse to take care of bathroom needs.

Paula talked about frequently awakening due to the difficulty of sleeping with paralysis. While we change positions unconsciously throughout the night, she had to awaken to consciously make these shifts. It took her some time to learn once again to sleep "normally."

The routines of daily life also differed significantly for Eileen and Carl. In the "old days" Carl woke up early, dressed, and left for the office. Now he would awaken late and Eileen needed to help him bathe, dress, and transfer to the wheelchair. Four days a week she drove him to the hospital for outpatient treatment. Afterwards, Carl would be so exhausted he would take a nap. On the days he did not have therapy, he rested in midday, returned to the wheelchair in the afternoon, and went to bed shortly after supper.

Paula's routine was established more quickly after her return home because her family was familiar with the type of care she needed. One of her parents helped transfer her to the wheelchair in the morning, where she then listened to her motivational tape at least twice and next practiced her physical therapy exercises. At lunchtime she returned to bed for a nap, then got up again at 1:00. She stayed up in her wheelchair until bedtime, often retiring as early as 7:00.

Julie was unable to reestablish her routines right away because "I was scared to death!" Although Ed was able to get around by himself, "I worried about him constantly!" This is not an unusual reaction. Julie had responded to the initial crisis because there was no choice; as life began to return to normal, some of her fear connected with the first weeks emerged and had to be dealt with. She found she couldn't sleep those first few nights until she accepted that nothing terrible was going to happen.

Ed didn't know what to do with himself at first, since his days used to be full of so many projects at the university. He found television too distracting because the words came too fast to make any sense. He tried turning the volume up and moving his chair closer to the set, but nothing seemed to help. His other favorite pursuit, reading, was too much effort to afford any relaxation. Julie enrolled him in the Talking Books program (see appendix: "Reading Materials for the Reader with Aphasia"), but Ed had some difficulty understanding because of the poor quality of the tapes and found buying taped books at a local bookstore more valuable.

In fact, there were so few things Ed could do independently that he wanted to be near Julie all the time, often following her from one room to the next. Because Ed had trouble "hearing" his own speech with the aphasia, he seemed to be talking and repeating himself constantly. Julie no longer had time to herself or for her hobbies. Although she loves Ed and feels spending time focusing on his recovery is crucial, this remains an area of conflict between them because her own needs are not being met. Discussing this issue together has helped, but since Ed's short-term memory was impaired as a result of the stroke, he often forgets the agreements he and Julie have made in their discussions. Time spent apart helps, Julie found, particularly at first, and visits from friends and relatives are a welcome relief to occupy Ed.

Resuming Activities and Responsibilities

Over time the stroke survivors and their families established new routines and life patterns. At first families assumed all household responsibilities in addition to caregiving, since it took time before the stroke survivor was able to help. We asked the families to share their memories of this transition, how they viewed the shift of roles, and what their reactions were when their family member began to try new things.

As Ed improved and his initial confusion abated, he began to want to do more. The first few times he went to get a haircut Julie accompanied him, but she soon decided that was needless. She could let him go alone, but to compensate for the difficulties he had with money concepts, she counted out the correct amount of money and tip before he left home. As Ed began shopping, going to the grocery store, and walking on his own, Julie's own early fears were reduced and Ed began to relax more, also.

Julie, like many other spouses, often worried that Ed's limited communication skills would be a problem if he ran into a difficult situation. To ease her fears, Ed carried a card put out by the American Heart Association explaining aphasia. The card included his name, address, phone, and emergency contact. Rehearsing ahead of time to prepare for new situations also helped. Families can role-play conversations with salespersons, waitresses, etc., to practice appropriate responses and to help the stroke survivor feel more confident with his communication.

Soon after his return home, Ed also wanted to get back to his office. Since he was not ready for work-related responsibilities, he and Julie decided that periodic visits would help him to reestablish necessary contacts with coworkers. Initially Julie drove him to campus and walked around with him as he visited. After the first year, Ed decided to ride the city bus since he could not drive yet because of his visual problems. This was a frightening new step for Julie—she knew Ed could manage in a familiar setting but realized that he could easily become disoriented in new places. To make herself more comfortable, she called the office about the time she estimated he should arrive, "just to check that he made it." One day Ed got lost when he caught the wrong bus home from the city. He, by this time, was able to keep calm despite the confusion, call his wife, and describe his surroundings well enough so that she could find him. Although she had worried something like this might happen, his response reminded her how far he had come in his recovery, and that she should continue to relax and allow his independence to blossom.

Eileen took complete responsibility for Carl during the first few months home. She acknowledges that other family members and friends would have been available for respite care, but she was too frightened to leave. She had to relinquish some control, however, when she realized that she had to get a job to provide needed income for the family. In retrospect, Eileen says it was most valuable to her husband's recovery and her own adjustment when she began working on Friday afternoons and Saturdays. As the days passed, she saw that Carl managed quite well for himself while she was at work. She became more confident in his ability to make decisions and handle new situations, and she watched as some of his previous fierce independence returned. For Carl, the responsibilities he now was forced to assume proved stimulating and aided his recovery. His self-confidence and pride in new accomplishments nourished him and created more energy and optimism when facing other challenges.

Gradually, even with his hemiparesis, Carl became more independent in his personal care. Because of his positive attitude and personality, he insisted on dressing, bathing, and grooming by himself. He also began to experiment with household tasks—an area that had been exclusively Eileen's before the stroke. As he got out of his wheelchair, Carl was able to straighten the house, vacuum, dust, wash dishes, fold laundry, and do some light cooking. Often he would surprise everyone with his creativity and ingenuity in the kitchen. One day he made an apple pie from scratch, peeling the apples with his one hand and following the recipe to assemble the crust and filling. Eileen, by now, was working full-time and asked Carl at one point if he would prefer that she stay home during the day. His response—an emphatic *"No!"* This arrangement provided both with needed space from one another, as well as an opportunity for Carl to increase his independence.

It took Ted about four months to emerge from his confusion and realize that "it was time to get on with my life." His fiftieth birthday party in March, 1985, stands out—a roaring success as his friends of so many years celebrated his birthday and his recovery. Realizing now that he had sole responsibility for his recovery, Ted began working again at his former company. He was sorting mail, a job that could "drive you cuckoo," but that nevertheless allowed him to feel productive and that he was a contributor to the family finances. His visual problems were so severe that he many times confused letters in a word or missed information at work, but he soon learned to compensate for these problems by scanning the writing more slowly. He also started helping Alice with the housework, bragging that his specialty was toilets.

Alice's memories of herself at this time are as "an appendage to Ted" once again. This time, of course, differed from the earlier period in their marriage, when they had sought counseling to help her regain her sense of independence. After working with a counselor in prior years to change their ways of relating to one another, it felt strange to be "locked together" once again. Alice began working full-time before Ted was well enough to also return to work. While she worried about leaving him alone, she reminded herself of his own need to redevelop independence. She still left work three days a week to drive Ted to his outpatient therapy, often so fatigued that she fell asleep while waiting for him. Nevertheless, during this time Alice became more confident in her abilities as the family's financial planner and decision-maker. She stresses how important it is that both partners have a clear understanding of the family finances in the event that something should happen to either one.

On many mornings Paula didn't even want to get out of

bed—overwhelmed by the tremendous energy it took just to do simple, ordinary tasks. She would remember her life before the illness, wondering, "why did I have to go through surgery and be left like this . . . why didn't they just let me go?" Yet she continued to push on, feeling that she must. Although she maintained this positive attitude most of the time, there were periods of depression, continuing physical pain, and lots of tears. Paula sought counseling with a psychologist intermittently throughout this period for added support. At times of great frustration when no words would come, she found relief by "just screaming!" Since her return home, Paula has found comfort time and again through loving and caring for her dog. She feels other stroke survivors might also gain pleasure from having a pet.

As Paula improved physically, she assumed the responsibility for self-care, as Carl had done. Her family worried about her increasing push to become more independent because early in her recovery she had taken a bad fall that set her back. When Paula's father took her to the bathroom one day she tried to stand alone, still lacking insight into her limitations. She fell against the vanity, breaking her front teeth. However, with time she regained her mobility. She graduated to using a cane and was fitted with a leg brace, always pushing to get better. One step to recovery was to stay alone at night. After two years of either one parent or the other spending the night, her mother was scared, wondering how Paula might handle various crises that might develop. Yet she and her husband withdrew in spite of their fears, allowing Paula to feel she had taken a giant step toward getting better. They hired a housekeeper half days to take care of household chores. Eventually, Paula was able to accomplish all her personal care, light housekeeping, and cooking. She has even entertained at her home, taking care of all the planning, shopping, and cooking. After she entertains, she is completely exhausted for a few days but says, "the feeling of accomplishment is worth it!"

Driving and Travel

Paula has resumed driving. Once again, her mother reflects on the fright that accompanied her joy and pride in seeing Paula regain an ability. She worried about rush-hour traffic and that the speed and irresponsibility of other drivers might cause an accident. But she had learned by now that the best way to handle this fear was to live through it, knowing that it would go away over time. This gain in independence was a tremendous boost for Paula. The ability to drive allowed her to once again feel a part of a society she felt she had been away from for a long time.

When Ed was stable enough to travel, the time came for him and Julie to decide whether to resume trips to their northern retreat. Julie had never driven on the expressway, but now she had to drive or they could not go. Although she was nervous, she chose to make the trip anyway and returned home with renewed self-confidence. Ed now drives, but with his limited visual field he knows that he needs to share the driving with his wife and that he cannot drive long distances as he used to before the stroke.

As Carl gained independence he, too, was ready to drive again. Eileen contacted an occupational therapy department that specialized in assessment of driving skills after strokes and arranged for him to receive a thorough evaluation. He was provided with adaptive equipment to accommodate his hemiparesis, a device to make steering easier, a left-foot accelerator, and training in how to use the new equipment. The evaluation also gave Eileen a chance to have her concerns addressed and to feel more comfortable with this next step.

Many stroke survivors, including those with paralysis, can drive again but often feel frightened about resuming this activity. Both families and stroke survivors concerned about safety issues can benefit from driver's evaluation and/or training. In instances where skills are sufficient, this provides the practice and support necessary to bolster confidence. If problems are noted, a class offers an opportunity for supervised training. Some may have to go through the evaluation more than once. In any case, the stroke survivor's first step before driving again is to talk to his primary physician. If he feels the stroke survivor is medically stable and grants permission to resume driving, it is often useful for the driver to practice first on a quiet street or in an empty parking lot. If the physician expresses concern about the patient's capability, a referral to a post-stroke driver's evaluation program, often offered through the occupational therapy department, is most appropriate.

Carl's brother, Allen, was nervous about his brother driving. Several thoughts raced through his mind: How would Carl ask for help while driving alone? How could he get gas without talking?

What would he do if he had a flat tire? Allen realized that his negative thinking contaminated Carl's determined, positive outlook. After reflecting on Carl's accomplishments so far, he reminded himself of the importance of his brother's need to continue to take risks and face new challenges. What was life without a struggle to improve? Allen realized this life process needed to occur regardless of the stroke. Carl had met risks before and was simply continuing as he always had, but now with a different set of variables. Allen could then focus his thoughts away from fear and toward love and pleasure, watching his brother's joy as he was able to do something constructive and useful.

Ted was not ready to drive again for two years. He felt that his vision on his right side was too limited and that traffic was too distracting. Since he moved about by walking or riding his bike, he didn't press himself to drive, figuring that he alone would know when he was ready. When Ted regained enough confidence he practiced first with his son. On one of his first times alone in the car, Ted encountered one road with two names where he was to turn. The person who had written the directions had jotted down the wrong name, and Ted ended up getting lost. Driving in a construction zone, he became more confused. He stopped at a gas station for directions, but the employees were too busy to write them out and Ted couldn't remember everything they said. Eventually he found his way out of the maze but returned home very defeated. After thinking about the situation, he decided that in the future instructions needed to be written down in more detail. Although his family was nervous as Ted started driving more each day, they realized the importance of "letting go," of allowing this next step to happen. In turn, Ted knows he will always have to be cautious because of his limited visual field, but he feels good about the return of this area of independence.

A frequently voiced concern is how and when travel should resume. Each of these families had enjoyed trips away from home before the stroke, either to a second home, favorite vacation spot, or to new areas. At the beginning of the illness and rehabilitation they felt hesitant to interfere with their newly established routines. While it is important not to interrupt rehabilitation, a trip can provide a time to relax and leave behind the thoughts of illness, to see the current situation from a different perspective.

Fatigue will always be a factor to anticipate in extended travel. Our families made sure to compensate for this in their itinerary before, during, and after travel. If an extended trip to another part of the country is important, rehabilitation programs would more than likely be available in that new location. Many said they were frightened to travel because of either their concern about handicapped facilities and/or fear of additional medical problems arising. They soon learned, however, that by anticipating their needs and calling to confirm handicapped access to restaurants and motels they avoided complications. Many agencies exist that can help the disabled traveler plan trips. Airlines can be called in advance to order a wheelchair when necessary. When traveling by car, frequent stops can be planned. While there is always the possibility of medical complications, good medical care should be available anywhere in this country. (In addition, most foreign countries have a list of medical resources for travelers.)

Over time families realize that worry about the "what ifs" interferes with the enjoyment of the trip. Each of these families found the more they traveled, the better "handicapped" travelers they became. As with other considerations associated with stroke recovery, the first time was the hardest; it became easier when some routines of traveling in this "new way" were established.

Associated Health Problems

After leaving the hospital for the last time, each person hoped his recovery would be free of any additional medical complications. Unfortunately that was not always the case. A common reaction in many families is continuing concern about other illness as well as fear of another stroke. While this is a realistic concern, because strokes caused by thrombi or emboli are indicative of vascular disease, it should also be said that the problem has been identified and medically managed; with the practice of good health habits (e.g., stopping smoking, exercising, and careful attention to diet), risk is reduced. Worry about additional medical complications is understandable considering the seriousness of the current problem, but this fear has to be put aside as much as possible so as not to interfere with living.

Alice and Lee both noted that their husbands were uncharacteristically cautious about their health, consulting their physicians at the first sign of any unusual symptom. Ted had difficulty with his bowels at first and after much experimenting had to change his diet. He attributes much of the problem, as he looks back on it, to the anxiety and frustration of the stroke. As he began running competitively again, he started seeing flashes of color in his head when he became too hot or fatigued. Needless to say he was frightened the first time this happened, but after consulting his physician, Ted determined that he was in no danger and was experiencing the symptoms because of the brain surgery. Since there are so few recorded case histories of individuals running competitively following a stroke, the symptoms were new to his doctor, yet considering Ted's excellent level of fitness, he felt this was more of an annoyance than a cause for concern.

Other setbacks that may occur following an insult to the brain are grand mal, petit mal, or focal seizures. A seizure involves a loss of control of body functioning of varying duration depending on its severity. While seizures are frightening to observe and uncomfortable for the stroke survivor to experience, they will not cause any additional damage to the brain. Only a minority of stroke survivors experience seizures. Some physicians elect to use anticonvulsant medication following a stroke to guard against this possibility. If a seizure should occur, it is advisable the first time to seek medical attention, as the doctor will need to determine a therapeutic dosage of anticonvulsant medication. It is not uncommon after a seizure for a person to feel very tired and to experience some reduction in his ability to communicate. The medication itself may cause drowsiness. Often several drugs and drug combinations may be used before determining the correct one. Blood levels will be checked while a person is medicated to establish a consistent therapeutic dosage. In some states it is required by law that, after a seizure, persons stop driving for a specified period of time.

Tom and Paula both have had seizures. The medical literature states that approximately 13 percent of those who have strokes resulting from embolus or thrombus have seizures; 90 percent of those seizures occur within two years after the stroke (Barnett 1986). Paula was put on an anticonvulsant medication immediately after surgery because of her previous history of seizures. It took time to find a therapeutic dosage for her, but when they did she was free of seizures for several years before suddenly experiencing them again. She would wake in the night sweating, dizzy, and unsure about what was happening. She did not consider seizure at first but was more concerned about another AVM. Her doctor increased her medication, but the seizures continued until she was too fatigued to participate in any of her outside activities. Finally, in desperation, she returned to her neurosurgeon, who experimented with changing the combination of the drugs, eventually controlling her seizures again.

Tom had his first seizure five months after his stroke. He was already so frustrated and discouraged that this intensified his depression. While at first the drugs would not control the seizures, his doctor found success after experimenting with a combination of anticonvulsant and antianxiety drugs. During this period Lee was encouraging Tom to become more independent by leaving him for longer periods by himself. But his anxiety about the possibility of more seizures caused him to become even more dependent for awhile. Any sensation of dizziness (sometimes an initial warning of a seizure) provoked many calls to Lee at work with the plea to come get him. Tom no longer has seizures, his period of dependency has ended, and he now drives again. He and his physician have been experimenting with ways to decrease the amount of his current medication to reduce his fatigue.

Financial Concerns

When the stroke occurs, attention is focused on the illness while other problems may be put aside to be dealt with later. As these families' lives resumed some semblance of normalcy, changes in the way they now lived together needed attention.

Carl and Eileen were faced with a major loss in income. Although Carl had health insurance to cover his medical expenses, he had no disability insurance and no income. Eileen was forced to sell the home they had built and their farm, their planned retirement home. She feels Carl handled this change better than she. Since she was apprehensive about dwelling on finances with a husband who already had so much to bear, she stressed the importance of moving to a single-story home where Carl wouldn't need to climb stairs. At first overwhelmed with business transactions she had never had to handle before, she gradually learned. From the start, Carl made it clear he wanted to be fully involved in the process of buying and selling his properties. He scanned the newspaper ads daily for homes and accompanied Eileen to look at selected ones. By this time Carl was walking with a cane, but he believes he would have gone with his wife even if he had still been confined to the wheelchair. By staying involved Carl was better able to cope with his sadness in moving, Eileen felt his support, and decisions could be shared.

About the time Carl returned from the hospital, it became more and more apparent that his company could not continue to operate without him. Carl had always carried primary responsibility as chief designer and engineer, and there was no one now to assume those duties. Eileen remembers the painful moment the family had to tell Carl his company would be sold. While at first he rejected the option, he eventually understood the necessity. Looking back upon this time, Carl's brother, Allen, feels that "the aphasia interfered with Carl's ability to get all the facts and fully comprehend the gravity of the situation." At first he was frustrated when Carl appeared to view very important issues with seeming nonchalance. Part of the problem for Carl was his inability to integrate all the facts. His brain just couldn't put together the different pieces of information he heard to get the whole concept. Carl ultimately got "enough pieces" to grasp the general idea of what needed to be done. His brother took him to the company shop for long hours of inventory and sorting equipment. Although he was sad over the loss of the company he had established and built, it was important for Carl to be an active participant in its dissolution. He seemed to gain a sense of control through involvement. Many stroke survivors have lost the opportunity for viable interaction at home and work, and this can be devastating to their egos. Feelings of powerlessness may be overwhelming. It is best to actively involve them, as Eileen did, in decision-making instead of protecting them from the difficulty and pain that result from necessary changes precipitated by the illness.

Adjustments in income were also a major issue for Paula. When she could no longer work, she at first received disability and unemployment income but was forced to use her savings when these benefits ran out. As her illness progressed, medical bills accumulated, giving her the added burden of worry over how she was going to meet her financial responsibilities. Now Paula receives federal disability. "It's been hard to have to change from being a saver, but I can't do that now." Paula had always enjoyed traveling both for business and pleasure, but trips, except short ones to stay with relatives, are financially out of the question now.

Ed and Julie also made financial adjustments. Both in their sixties, they had money saved and were more financially secure than younger couples may be who experience a stroke. Julie did not have to get a job but did so for reasons other than financial. About a year after his stroke, Ed was away from home a few days a week at his office. Julie was depressed because so much of her life during the past year had been devoted to her husband and his needs. When she realized she was withdrawing from others because of her sorrow and pain, she found a part-time job to increase her involvement with others again.

Alice and Lee continued to work full-time, taking only a brief time away from their jobs during the acute stages of the illness. They had young families, with some children in school and others planning for or currently in college. Alice enjoyed the freedom of working and making her own money but this was a difficult transition for Ted, who was used to being the chief provider and manager of family investments and finances. Since the family now relied solely on her income, it felt strange for Ted to watch his children go to his wife for money. Alice at first knew nothing about paying bills, so when one came she would panic and pay it immediately; now she has learned to manage the checkbook and has become more relaxed and confident about money management.

Social Considerations

The opportunity for socialization after stroke is often lessened. During the acute stages of illness, when physical healing and outpatient rehabilitation are priorities, stroke survivors and their families feel isolated socially. Friends often fade from the picture, perhaps not aware how much continued support is needed. Family members may hesitate to express a need for support, fearing that they may be a burden to their friends. When routines have been established after the return home and stroke survivors and their families begin to seek social stimulation, they are often surprised and disappointed by the reaction of others.

Friendships changed for Julie and Ed, as they did for each of the families in this book. Julie neither fully understands nor accepts why people now ignore them. While a few friends have continued to help them through the hard times, she hurts to see her husband ignored at social events because he is now less capable of starting a conversation.

It took two years for Paula to regain sufficient energy and confidence to begin going out again. She developed enough speech over time to feel that she was now able to get her point across in a conversation and with improved communication she felt more comfortable with the risk of interacting with strangers, who might respond in ways that hurt. When she and her mother went to a restaurant one day, she remembers the looks and grimaces from other patrons as the hostess led them to their table. Feeling self-conscious because of the stares, Paula and her mother were finally seated, only to see the people next to them make it clear they were going to get up and leave. Paula's mother recalls her own pain and anger: "We come up against these kinds of situations . . . and I almost wish they could take her place for a week . . . people don't understand." Paula learned quickly that most other people responded with little patience, especially for her slow speech, so she started using phrases such as "Wait a minute," or "I'm trying" to slow others down and keep them from rushing her. When she meets new people she prefers to let them do the talking. "I say, 'how are you doing?', then I shut my mouth and listen!"

Paula had also lost the support of her women friends. Even though she had a fairly expansive social network, most women her age were frightened by Paula's experience with illness and her difficulty with communication. They did not know how to relate to her and so ignored her. Paula feels most had second thoughts or felt badly—she remembers hearing many excuses. But she understood what the excuses really meant. It was hard to know that people she cared about were viewing her as "weird" and to lose these supports at a time when she was experiencing so many other losses.

Yet, over time, the hurt has lessened. "Anymore, I don't feel so bad. I am me. They thought I should be well—that even though I was Paula, I couldn't be the person they used to know. I am the same person." Most of Paula's close friendships now are with other disabled persons. She finds greater support and acceptance from them—it's all right for her to have aphasia. She can relax, have fun, and take her time communicating with them.

After coming home, then, it is important to begin reentry into social activities so as to avoid focusing totally on illness. New supports might be found in stroke clubs or other previously unexplored avenues. At this time of transition, it is valuable to assess your current needs, since they may have changed, and then carefully plan ways to meet them. Most of these families now feel an increasing need for types of support that provide love and intimacy, guidance and comfort, as well as new stimulation and challenge.

Return to Exercise

Many stroke survivors wonder about resuming physical exercise and/or recreational pursuits after returning home. It is advisable first to check with a physician, physical therapist, recreational therapist, and/or exercise physiologist, who can advise as to when and how exercise can begin. Physical fitness is as important now as before, but often many are hesitant to begin because of a hemiparesis or concern about another stroke. When they do, stroke survivors say it not only increases their level of fitness and flexibility, but it helps them relax and feel better about themselves as well. For those with a residual hemiparesis, physical exercise can prevent atrophy of the remaining muscles. Re-establishing recreational pursuits is equally important. Instruction that focuses on new ways to pursue a favorite sport can help a person learn to compensate for any limitations in mobility.

Soon after his return home, each stroke survivor posed the question about exercise and how much was "safe." Ed was aware of his weight gain, so he decided to begin walking on a regular basis. Although he became exhausted quickly when he started, he slowly gained stamina. As he began feeling stronger, he decided to try to cross-country and downhill ski, sports he had loved before. His physician urged moderation, and Ed felt his body would let him know when he had had enough. Returning to sports that had given him so much pleasure was exhilarating, but his body, even without the hemiparesis, did feel "different." He did not seem as rhythmic and had a difficult time on the ski slopes executing turns toward his affected right side. With practice this improved, but he was aware that his stamina was now reduced.

Betty felt so sluggish that she started swimming three days a week through a program with her stroke club. The first step was overcoming a new fear of the water. Since her right side was paralyzed, she wasn't sure she would still float. One of the volunteers showed her how buoyant the body is by tying his feet and arms together, jumping in the pool and "bobbing" in the water. Betty gradually was able to swim lengths of the pool and then, wearing weights, use the resistance of the water to strengthen her entire body. At first she was lowered into the pool with a special lift, but now she jumps in at the deep end. (Often, though stroke survivors can see the benefits of water exercise, they don't swim because the water feels too cold. This is a valid concern; before participating in a swim program, Betty had to find a pool that maintained a constant warm-water temperature.) Betty also missed golf and took lessons to learn how to swing a club with her left arm only. In her case, while she has learned to hit the ball, one of her persistent problems is keeping up with play because of the extra time needed to get in and out of the golf cart. (Many stroke survivors who only have use of one arm have learned to play golf successfully by using specially weighted irons that are shorter and equipped with a larger grip. Some who do not have a residual hemiparesis and can use both hands still find problems with balance and weight shift as they swing a golf club.)

Before his stroke, Tom took pride in his athletic prowess, so his loss of agility took time to manage. As he got out of his wheelchair, he began experimenting with ways to continue the sports he had enjoyed before his stroke. He now bowls by stepping up to the alley before throwing the ball. He played golf with his left arm only but found, as Betty did, that the golf courses were so busy he had difficulty keeping up with the people ahead of him. To keep his exercise program varied, he began swimming at a local pool and exercising with weights three times a week. Eventually Tom began to walk for exercise and recently completed a ten-mile walk for a local charity with only occasional use of his wheelchair. Tom also tried wheelchair basketball but found it too much of a challenge using only one arm.

Paula also has entered walking competitions with other disabled individuals sponsored by local recreation departments. At first she walked in shopping malls where the climate was controlled and the surfaces were even. Participation in handicapped aerobics helped Paula increase her fitness level. Programs like this, when supervised by trained therapists, are excellent ways to maintain flexibility and also may provide good social outlets.

Ted found his need for exercise returning as the weakness on the right side of his body eased. Although he spends most of his time in competitive running, he found use of the rowing machine and stationary bike important to his training. Eventually he started biking outdoors once again. Many stroke survivors who have a persistent hemiparesis find they can still enjoy outdoor cycling by using a three-wheeled bicycle built especially for adults.

Conclusion

Coming home from the hospital, then, is a step full of emotional and physical transitions. Over the first few weeks and months, facing one new situation after another can be very taxing on all participants. Until new routines are in place, the stress associated with making guesses about what is the "right" thing to do in any given situation can be exhausting. Keeping up with full schedules, which include doctor's appointments, treatment sessions in rehabilitation, and daily care, is not an easy task. It is a time when finding ways to rest, people to talk to, and a "shoulder to lean on" are important and necessary parts of living.

Families soon learn the importance of fitting their own wants and needs into time that might be otherwise totally absorbed by the needs of the stroke survivor. The family member who has had the stroke can easily lose perspective of his own progress in this painfully slow process of moving away from "what used to be" toward "getting better." Rejoicing with one another when signs of improvement are noticed helps fuel the motivation of all involved. Sharing progress gives reassurance that all are doing the best they can no matter what their efforts.

Experimenting with different ways to do "old things" or ways to try "new things" can be fun if the healing power of humor is remembered. When Ed couldn't recognize his toe poking through his sock, he and Julie turned it into a moment for laughter instead of awkwardness and estrangement from each other. After rehabilitation sessions, Alice and Ted often laughed as he attempted to say something that just somehow didn't come out the "right" way. These families had started the necessary process of "letting go of illness" as they began their journey toward resuming life once again.

4.

Aphasia: Loss of Communication

Loss of communication was one of the most difficult changes each family faced. None had ever considered this possibility; most had never even heard the word "aphasia," a derivitive of the Greek word, *aphatos*, meaning "not speak." Over time they realized aphasia did not mean the loss of all language competence but only that to some degree, different with everyone, ability to use language symbols was now reduced.

It is difficult for most to understand this language loss, for it is complex. There is no simple way to explain the subtle and abstract functions our brain performs as we communicate. In fact, like breathing and walking, it is an "automatic" ability we rarely think about until something happens to interrupt it. With the stroke, all six families suddenly had to discover the process of normal communication in order to realize what skills their family member had lost. Our families came to realize that brain injury sometimes means that certain brain centers can no longer resume their previous function. Nonetheless, communication can and does improve over a longer period of time, as other brain centers take over the function or develop new ways to accomplish the lost function.

When brain centers are not injured so severely, they can recover. Early on, the severity of the illness itself makes it impossible to determine how much communication will return. The trauma to the brain tissue causes it to swell and chemical changes interfere with the workings of the healthy tissue surrounding the ischemic (dead) brain tissue. As the majority of the edema (swelling) subsides in the first month to six weeks, communication will steadily improve. (All the cerebral edema, however, may not subside for six months to a year.)

So, in effect, some communication returns spontaneously, some returns through treatment as brain centers learn new functions, and some losses may remain as residuals of the stroke. Even this residual loss can often be successfully managed through treatment centered on ways to compensate for it, as we will explain later. Ted, Betty, Tom, Ed, Carl, and Paula all recovered communication. Although they communicate differently now, they can successfully interact with family, friends, and strangers.

Our families learned about aphasia by reading about it, experimenting with communicating at home, and working with a speech and language pathologist in treatment. We are often asked what speech and language treatment involves and if it is really useful, since problems don't seem to disappear after a few treatment sessions. Rather than as a clinician who restores communication, the speech and language pathologist serves as a resource to explain what areas of the brain are deficient and to devise and implement exercises to help enable the compensatory process to happen. Our families found that the speech and language pathologist shared suggestions about how to communicate with stroke survivors who could no longer talk, write, read, and understand as they had before.

Problems with Listening: Auditory Comprehension

Imagine yourself a stranger in a foreign land. You perceive the environment surrounding you, understanding the universality of blue sky, land, mountains, buildings, faces, movement, and music. Yet you cannot comprehend the language that is spoken. Sound registers and lips move; you understand that people are talking with intent to communicate. You struggle to interpret—concentrate, watch, and welcome any recognizable word. Those who raise their voices in an effort to help your struggle for understanding distract you—speech that was at first nonsense now becomes noise. And those who speak too quickly tax your concentration and "overload" you. But those who watch carefully for signs that you have understood, who point and gesture, who may even use pictures, and who pace their words more slowly become those you understand best.

This can be the world to the stroke survivor. Nearly all those with aphasia have some degree of an auditory comprehension problem. Roberta Chapey (1986), in *Language Intervention Strategies in Adult Aphasia,* defines auditory comprehension problems as "impairments in assigning meaning to incoming auditory messages or to understanding words as they relate to objects, persons, ideas and experience." In other words, the stroke survivor loses ability, to some degree, to understand a simple spoken word like "chair," verbal directions like "Get the mail, please," statements like "I think the new Taurus is a reliable car," television, movies, or an amusing story. When a person having this problem fails to connect words with their correct meanings he may respond in a variety of ways: inappropriately, blankly, confusedly, silently, quizzically, by signaling that he doesn't understand, or by changing to another subject. Because "comprehension" is not a visible process, lack of it can easily be misinterpreted as a loss of intelligence. But the aphasic's response, or absence of it, is not an indication of a lack of knowledge. On the contrary, the aphasic individual knows very well what a chair is, how to get the mail, and how people share insights through exchanging comments, stories, and jokes. It is the inability of the brain to perform this associative function, connecting word to meaning, that is the problem in aphasia.

Think of a lamp with a cord that has a short circuit. The power source is intact; the bulb is good; yet the lamp works efficiently some of the time and not at all at other times because the connecting pathway to conduct the current is damaged. Similarly, connecting pathways in the brain between auditory centers and other centers that store the vocabulary we have learned are damaged by a stroke. Once the nature of this auditory problem is understood, it is easier to see that the aphasic person is still thinking as an adult, not a child. The cerebral "light bulb" is still intact. He remains aware of life around him, has opinions, feelings, and thoughts just as before.

Nearly all persons with aphasia have some difficulties understanding what they hear, but the degree of this comprehension problem varies considerably. Affecting factors can include the severity of the stroke, the particular location of damage in the brain, and the degree of any existing hearing loss. A severe stroke might compromise a person's ability to understand television, conversation, simple words, and all but very short yes or no questions, whereas a mild stroke may only reduce his ability to gain full meaning from humorous stories, innuendo, and lengthy, involved directions. Everyone with aphasia should be thoroughly evaluated by a speech and language pathologist to determine the degree of auditory comprehension difficulties and to learn appropriate ways to manage them.

The aphasic person may not realize when he is failing to understand a spoken message and that is why he may not ask to have it repeated or explained. In general, the more severe the aphasia, the less likely the person is to be aware of his comprehension difficulties. Betty, Paula, Tom, Carl, Ed, and Ted all reported believing shortly after their stroke that "everyone else was confusing" them. They could neither interpret what others were saying to them nor monitor (listen to) their own speech as they were talking. All of us normally monitor ourselves as we speak, although we are seldom conscious of doing so. As we hear our own words a part of our brain "checks out" what we are saying. A signal is sent that we need to make a correction if the message sounds wrong. We then might typically add more to the message, revise our wording, or start over. Persons with aphasia who cannot monitor their own words lose this vital feedback loop.

To further illustrate, imagine you suddenly lost your ability to hear. Aside from not being able to hear others, you can no longer hear your own voice. The act of speaking would become more of a guess—you would form words by "feel." You would also lose awareness of how loud you were speaking, what your vocal tone was like, or whether you were pronouncing words correctly. Perhaps you would have a memory of what your speech used to sound like that was different from how it actually sounded. For example, Ed often thought his own words came out exactly as they were planned in his head, when in fact they were completely different. Over time, as the auditory problem lessened and he relearned to monitor in treatment, he began to hear and revise his own words.

Obviously, problems in auditory comprehension can profoundly affect conversational exchange, for the ability to gain meaning from listening is basic to communication. When the aphasic person misunderstands, his response may be inappropriate and the conversation breaks down. In more subtle instances, the speaker and the listener will walk away from a conversation thinking the communication was successful but with totally different impressions. We are all aware of how this happens on a day-to-day basis: person A swears person B never said X, while person B is convinced he did. With auditory comprehension difficulties this very common problem occurs more often. It is crucial to consider this when communicating with the aphasic person so that misunderstandings are not taken personally.

In order to fully understand the difficulties, it is helpful to learn about the different levels of impairment and associated problems.

Attention

Aphasia may cause changes in attention. The auditory system may fail, or inconsistently "activate" to the sound of spoken words. You may find yourself talking to a person who is not even aware you are speaking. This can be the root of misunderstandings because the nonaphasic individual is sure that "I already told him that." To minimize this, it may help to say the person's name, touch him, or get his attention in some way before giving the message.

Once attention is established it may not always remain consistent. Aphasia causes changes in the brain's ability to sustain attention to sound, especially for long periods and particularly when the individual is fatigued. It takes a great amount of intentional concentration for the aphasic person to compensate for this problem. You need to watch for signs that attention is drifting, take breaks when this happens, and help redirect the individual back to the exchange. This attention will be difficult to attain in situations with background noise. A television or radio playing in the same room, a group of people talking at a party, or the noise of a crowded restaurant can be extremely distracting for the aphasic person, and his ability to focus auditory attention on one conversation becomes exhausting and nearly impossible. It is best to eliminate these distractions, limit the amount of time in these situations, and save more important information to communicate in a quieter place.

Auditory-Verbal Agnosia

In more severe cases of aphasia, an auditory-verbal agnosia may interfere with understanding. Here, agnosia refers to an inability to attach meaning to spoken words. It occurs primarily with nouns and names but can also limit understanding of verbs, adjectives, adverbs, and numbers. The aphasic may keep repeating an unfamiliar word after he hears it in an attempt to feed the sound back into his auditory system in order to trigger recognition. Or he may respond inappropriately (e.g., bring a plate instead of a fork to the direction, "Hand me that fork, please") because a "short circuit" occurred the brain associated the wrong meaning with the word. When this happens, awareness of it varies. There are times when the individual is very concerned by his lack of word recognition, and times when he will have no idea of his mistake. In this instance putting the word in context can provide more information to the brain. Instead of saying, "Hand me that fork," it is better to say, "Hand me the fork, the one with the points," gesture, and/or write the word. Like a computer, the brain responds better when more information is added, enabling faster and more accurate word recognition.

Comprehending Sentences

Another level of understanding occurs when we listen to phrases and sentences. Normally, we hear a group of words together in a sentence, and our brain automatically performs a complex function of getting meanings for each individual word plus putting them all together to understand the entire message. "Since dinner is at 8:00 we'll go to the 9:30 show" is entirely different from "We'll go to the show at 8:00 since dinner is at 9:30."

The person with auditory comprehension problems loses some ability to interpret these word relationships. His auditory center is no longer automatically getting word meanings and comparing and associating them to get the full message. For a moment reconsider our discussion of visiting a foreign country where you have no knowledge of the language. This time, however, let's assume that you have taken some language courses. As you listen to those persons trying to communicate with you, you now recognize a few words in each sentence. Suppose someone says, "If you take the second right you will find the restaurant you are looking for." As you listen, you understand the words "right" and "restaurant." You put these words together and assume you turn right at the next corner to get to the restaurant. Because you missed the important word "second" in the sentence, you failed to understand the message completely; although you probably *thought* you understood, you missed the main point.

Generally, the more abstract the message of a sentence, the more unusually worded, and the more complicated its grammatical form, the harder it will be for the aphasic person to interpret reliably. Some word relationships difficult for the person with aphasia to interpret include: prepositions (above, behind, on); comparative terms (bigger, older than, latest); words relating to time concepts (before, after); negatives and contractions; and conditional terms (if——then——). (For a more complete list, refer to the appendix, "Language Difficulties for the Aphasic Affecting Reading.") The constructions described there are also difficult when spoken. When giving directions or conversing, it is best to simplify language to make verbal messages straightforward and concrete.

Retention

A stroke survivor with reduced auditory comprehension nearly always experiences changes in retention abilities. This refers to the capability to "hold in our heads" or remember what we have heard immediately after hearing it. This is sometimes referred to as "short-term memory" ability. Normally, this is an automatic function that we use daily, as illustrated by our capability to remember a phone number, respond to directions, or recall a story. A person who has had a stroke with aphasia can't remember the amount of information he did before. Now when hearing a phone number he may only "hold in his head" two of the numbers—and thus be unable to repeat it or write it down, much less dial it. Many times the memory for the first part of a message fades before its completion. The person may hear a news story on television, and by the end of the broadcast forget what it was about. Retention ability is vital to our thinking process—we listen to, then mentally review and juggle pieces of information to form conclusions. If all the information doesn't stick, our perceptions and conclusions will be altered. To the person with aphasia this difficulty occurs constantly. Compensatory strategies can be useful in minimizing the frustration this causes the aphasic and making him feel more capable. If the person can read, provide information in writing in addition to saying it. Find out the limits of his retention span and adjust your message to fit this. Don't give him four things to remember if he can only handle two. If the person can write, encourage him to take notes as he listens.

Integration

Limited comprehension for stories, jokes, puns, innuendo, and subtle messages is also characteristic of auditory impairment. At this level the brain must recognize word meaning, interpret the grammatical form of the message, retain the facts, and pull this information together to conclude. Putting facts together, or "integrating information," as this function is known, is reduced. When the stroke patient's impairment is mostly in this auditory area the difficulty is not as obvious to others. Those communicating with him experience communication breakdown less frequently. Therefore it is easy to assume appropriate comprehension has taken place. To illustrate, imagine for a moment that I have a problem integrating facts and listen to you tell me the following joke. "Yesterday I went down to the boat show to see the latest models. My favorite was the yacht with this sign inside: 'The shower door has been removed for your viewing pleasure.'"

I listen, and understand that you went to the boat show, thought it was fun, and liked the one with the pretty bathroom. You laugh, and I laugh with you. We have shared communication; you assume I "got" the joke and I assume I "got" the story. I walk away never realizing the play on words. Although I heard your words, I was unable to interpret them beyond a concrete level. If I happen to be aware of how my auditory comprehension difficulties affect my listening, I might sense I had missed something and ask you to explain the joke. Generally, however, the stroke survivor at this level is not likely to be aware that he has missed the point since he is getting a real message. This type of impairment can cause communication problems in intimate relationships when indirectly worded messages are taken literally, causing misunderstandings. Once again, it is helpful to manage this problem by becoming more aware of how it can affect both the aphasic person and the family. When misunderstanding occurs, the possibility of the auditory comprehension difficulty as a factor can be explored.

Additional Factors

So far we have defined an auditory comprehension problem and examined the different levels of impairment: difficulties in attention, auditory-verbal agnosia, reduced ability to comprehend sentences, and decreased retention and integration skills. These levels are not clearcut in that more than one is involved in nearly all cases, particularly as the severity increases. There are also other characteristics associated with auditory comprehension problems of which we must be aware.

With aphasia, the brain "interprets" information at a slower rate, and the stroke survivor needs extra time when listening before the message makes sense. Thus continuous messages, especially when given at a fast rate, will result in "overload"— similar to overloading an electrical circuit. The brain, in effect, can't keep up with this constant feed of information and shuts down processing. We all experience this auditory overload from time to time, but the threshold for its occurrence is significantly lower for the person with aphasia. Now he may have trouble just hearing the whole television newscast or a movie. Some may be frustrated, some may pretend disinterest, while others may just walk away: the response differs for everyone. It is useful to find out what each person's tolerance is and learn what the signs of overload are. Take breaks when overload occurs and save important information to be reviewed later. In some cases, as the aphasic person learns to recognize when overload begins to occur, he can exert more control of the communication by signaling his own need to stop.

Similarly, the auditory system often needs additional "warm-up" time, also called "slow rise." A cold copying machine will not make copies immediately after being turned on, yet a few minutes later systems are ready to operate. With the aphasic person signs of this need to "warm up" can be a persistent lack of comprehension irrespective of how the message is simplified or shortened. This is followed by a period when the "light bulb" goes on—the person begins to comprehend these same messages he was unable to grasp a few minutes before. This phenomenon does not occur only at the beginning of the day or in the first few minutes of a conversation. It can occur several times throughout the day or when conversation shifts to a new topic. Again, minimizing the effects means trying to increase your awareness of when "slow rise" is happening. Although you cannot stop it, you can help the aphasic person through a warm-up period by using casual social speech, saving the gist of your message until he is best able to make sense out of the information. When switching subjects, allow extra time for the shift. Sometimes it is necessary to take a short break or to stop the conversation entirely.

Because the auditory centers are interpreting information more slowly in general, it is important to adjust your speaking rate when communicating with an aphasic person. You should not speak abnormally slowly, because this will interrupt the rhythm of the language, causing added confusion. Instead, keep the natural pauses in your message, but hold them slightly longer. Stop after each sentence to allow interpretation before going on. Experiment with different speaking rates to find the best one. Even if the person cannot decode the word meanings in the question, "Do you think we should stop at Ann's before going home?" he will know you are asking something due to the rising intonation of your voice at the end of the sentence. Again, this is why someone with severe auditory problems can look like he is understanding the conversation. Pleasure, anger, frustration, sadness— all are communicated in vocal tone at the same time as we are expressing it in words. If the intonation of our speech does not fit with the verbal message, confusion can result. The aphasic person relies a great deal on the intonation he hears to assist him in processing messages. Thus it is important to retain normal intonation in your voice as you talk. Although a slight exaggeration in such intonation is sometimes appreciated, it is unwise to exaggerate too much. This is distracting and results in a feeling of being "talked down to" and generally treated like a child. By the same token, it is important to retain normal loudness when speaking.

Experiences of Stroke Survivors and Their Families

What does all this feel like to the person experiencing it? Betty, Paula, Carl, Ted, Tom, and Ed shared their impressions.

When Betty was in the hospital she always wanted to hear information a second time. Although she was aware she needed this, she didn't find it unusual at the time and never connected it with a change in her auditory system because of aphasia. This awareness did not come until later, as she improved and worked with her speech and language pathologist to learn the nature of her stroke-induced aphasia. Early on, she assumed her need for redundancy was the speaker's problem, that some people were just better talkers than others, and she found herself irritated with those who spoke fast and were "poor expressors." As she has improved, she is now often aware when her auditory system is processing inefficiently. In many cases, particularly early on when auditory comprehension impairments are at their worst, blankness, frustration, anger, or indignation can be signs that the person with the aphasia is not aware of his problem and feels that those around him are just trying to be confusing.

Tom found himself more argumentative at first. He, as well as Ed and Paula, vividly remembers hearing echoes and ringing in his ears, distracting him as he tried to listen. Although this lasted for some time it eventually faded away, unrelated to any hearing abnormality. Tom is aware that when he is tired he "just can't get" messages. Nearly everyone felt fluctuations in their auditory system, particularly with fatigue. Some days are just bad days with no seeming explanation, and some are good. This may lessen somewhat with time but usually becomes a factor to manage for a lifetime.

Ed felt constant confusion in what he heard while on the rehabilitation floor. His first breakthrough remains a special memory for him: he recognized his own words being spoken by his speech and language pathologist, who was reading from one of Ed's published books. It helped to hear what was familiar to him. After that, comprehension was not consistent, but was characterized by on and off periods of awareness. Because Ed had previously spoken several foreign languages, his sensitivity to anything he heard that was strange or unrecognizable was heightened. He tended to assume the person was speaking in a foreign language he was not familiar with. He remembers asking persons in rehabilitation, "What language are you speaking?" He recalls his struggle and confusion with this at one point when he was getting a CT scan and couldn't understand the verbal directions of the technicians. (Directions are nearly always a problem for persons with auditory difficulty because the information is so specific. A sentence of conversation is much easier to follow than a sentence of instruction.) Presently, Ed is more aware of his reduced comprehension and asks people to repeat messages as necessary. He has particular difficulty with words related to size, shape, and color concepts and uses other senses, such as smell, to help him associate meanings. He is now able to listen to his own classroom lectures by tape-

recording his rehearsals and evaluating the effectiveness and organization of his speech as he reviews them.

Carl found it easiest to understand his wife at first, relying
heavily upon her communication with him early in his recovery.
Stroke survivors often understand spouses and family members
better than others because vocal tone, intonation patterns, facial
expressions, and mannerisms are so well known. Also, a family
member often has an intuitive ability to modify messages in a
manner the stroke survivor understands. Eileen often became
Carl's "translator." Today, Carl has most trouble understanding
those who speak too loudly and too fast.

Paula spent her first year after surgery hating loud noises,
finding them overwhelming to her auditory system. She felt best
when she was alone because of her inability to understand what
she was hearing. She believes she was not aware of the auditory
deficit for some time. Looking back, she felt angry and bewildered. "I didn't know what I was supposed to do." She smiled a lot
to others in spite of her confusion in an effort to feel included and
participate "normally." Constant acknowledgment of her lack of
understanding would have been overwhelming. (The aphasic person may smile, nod, and generally give the false impression he
comprehends at times, as this enables him to experience the natural flow of communicative exchange. We gain closeness, com-
munion, and pleasure from this rhythm in and of itself, and it is
perfectly appropriate to allow the aphasic person the opportunity
to share in this way.) When Paula found her auditory comprehension skills improving, she gradually became able to tolerate more
exposure to crowds. Previously, she had avoided restaurants, parties, and family gatherings and now feels groups of three to four
persons are ideal for conversation, although she has to concentrate to tune out other noises. She is also able to enjoy television
again. What was once fast and distracting is now comprehended,
but only for limited periods of time.

Ted is amused as he thinks of episodes when he misinterpreted information. A year after his stroke he proudly went to
his first baseball game alone but he didn't give the ticket agent
the correct amount of money because the numbers "sounded
alike." And later he drank his way through three large Cokes after
he failed to hear his own misspoken words when ordering them.
Now he looks for visual cues to assist him in his understanding.
When making purchases, he watches the cash register to see the

total amount. And he finds that if he can see a word as a person says it, he will understand better. When he first started driving again, he had to have the car radio turned off; now he has gradually allowed outside noises back in without compromising comprehension but still "overloads" easily. To him, "It's not a hearing loss . . . you can hear . . . it just sounds like things are going too fast."

While these are some of the feelings stroke survivors may have, how does an auditory problem seem to the persons living closest to them? We asked the spouse and family members to discuss their perceptions and learnings, and to share insights about coping with auditory deficits. All agreed that this area of impairment is one of the hardest to understand. Again, because comprehension is not visible, it is an abstract concept to explain or perceive. Most spouses felt that they had false impressions of the degree of information their partner was actually able to understand at first, that there was some degree of denial on their part in accepting this was actually happening, and that it took them a long time to realize the nature and extent of the difficulty. It is a continual learning process to develop sensitivity in detecting when auditory problems interfere in communication and to learn how to manage them.

Julie sensed her husband's lack of understanding right away because his problem was so severe. His inappropriate responses or lack of responses were obvious indications that little information was actually getting through to him. She quickly learned how to use repetition. It was very important to Julie that her husband still feel a part of what was going on about him, so she did not stop telling him things even though she knew he was not understanding much of it. Early on it became common practice to repeat information five or more times. Now, even though she may only need to do this two or three times, repetition is still a tedious process. Most spouses feel it disrupts communicative flow—the "easy" exchange, the intimate, light banter that bonds the relationship and creates a couple's "comfort zone." With this flow gone, an important part of good communication is missing.

As Ed's auditory deficits have improved, his ability to monitor his own speech and to be aware of his lack of understanding has increased. At one point in his recovery he could watch TV and realize that he had missed some information. Ed tried to repeat this immediately or ask Julie to repeat it in an attempt to feed it back through his auditory system before he lost the con-

cept. But for Julie this was highly disruptive. She found less opportunity to watch a program completely without having to stop and
repeat parts of it to her husband. Although she knew this was a
sign of improvement, she had a greater communicative burden as
long as Ed relied on translation and explanation from her. Ultimately this behavior disappeared as Ed became more able to process information directly from the television.

Alice also finds this explanation and repetition exhausting.
At times, she feels herself interacting as she did when parenting
small children. Extra time must be taken to review, give examples, and simplify language—and still sometimes these interactions end in frustration. She misses the opportunity to have a
"normal," automatic exchange with her husband. Alice has found
some compensation in conversing with her son, but this has been
difficult for Ted, as he would cherish such "normal" conversation
with his wife and would prefer to be the one providing it for her.
Couples may feel conflicting feelings when the aphasic person,
though he may understand his spouse's need for conversing with
other adults, still feels resentment. Although Ted no longer has
the capability to carry on an "easy" conversation, he still has the
desire to do so. The spouse, on the other hand, may feel guilty
about wanting and needing communication with others, yet
needing to protect the stroke survivor from further hurt. It can
help to discuss these conflicting emotions as a couple, realizing
that each is a perfectly normal response to the situation.

Alice also finds it difficult to cope with others' interpreta-
tions of her husband's comprehension problems. It is hard for her
to hear friends question Ted about what he understands or to
misconstrue his level of intellectual awareness. As Ted's comprehension has improved, Alice finds she can now repeat his mistakes to him so that he can hear them and, at times, correct them.
Since it would be overwhelming to Ted for her to do this all the
time, she sometimes "lets it go." Alice also finds phone conversations particularly hard since Ted needs repetition and extra time
to organize his own responses. Phone calls from work, for example, usually need to be made in the shortest time possible. She
feels pressured by the conflict between Ted's need for delay to
interpret what she says and her own responsibility to keep up
with the pace at work.

Carl's brother remembers his early reactions to Carl's auditory difficulties: "Despite a communication problem, we all
believed that he was aware of what we were telling him . . . then

at times, we were completely and utterly dismayed at the lack of communications." Eileen, after initially hearing the strange word "aphasia," gradually learned the extent of the auditory problem. She always felt that Carl understood her best, realizing that the issues they discussed were very familiar to them both. When Carl first returned home, she remembered him turning off the car radio as they drove, and his going in another room to be by himself in the middle of a family Christmas celebration, something he never would have done before the stroke. It took time to realize this was his way of managing auditory overload and distraction. Eileen compensates for any reductions in retention or problems interpreting directions by leaving short written notes for Carl. Thus he sees as well as hears the message and doesn't have to expend extra concentration trying to remember it. Eileen now is able to call Carl from work. Because his speech is limited, she adjusts her questions so they can be answered by "yes" or "no." Although Carl hated the television at first, she has seen him return to his old habits of watching movies or shows for hours. Carl's son and his family were distressed about how to communicate an idea at first, but over time have experimented with trial and error, "charade" clues, twenty questions, pictures, and other ways besides verbal messages of getting information to the brain.

When Paula was in the rehabilitation unit, her mother thought she was much more aware than she later discovered. At one point she found it helpful when her doctor explained that Paula only *looked* as if she understood but was actually taking in very little information. It has been hard for her brother to see old friends abandon Paula, misinterpreting her difficulty with comprehension as a loss of her intelligence. Soon after her surgery he found himself guessing how much of what he said was understood. He wondered at the time how he could help make it easier and recalls his initial, unintentional tendency to talk more slowly and loudly. Now he finds rephrasing is more effective in getting a point across.

Lee finds her husband reacting to information differently than he used to. It is impossible for her to predict his reaction to information now, whereas prior to the stroke she could have guessed his responses. In this case, although changed attitudes could be a factor, it is quite likely that Tom's comprehension difficulties lead to altered perceptions of messages at times. Judgment appears different and he seems to lack insight because of his inability to grasp all of the information. Some persons may assume this is due to expressive difficulties, personality change, behavioral reactions, or loss of intellectual ability in the aphasic patient. The possibility of even mild auditory comprehension problems causing changes should be explored and discussed with spouses and families.

Lee is also learning to live with a husband who now forgets things easily. Since he can't retain as much information just as he hears it, messages are not stored as efficiently in his long-term memory. Socially, he is often excluded in conversation with friends. Because of the extra time he needs to interpret what he hears others say, he often cannot respond as quickly. As long as a period of silence follows the delivery of the message Tom is able to follow what is being said, but in group conversation periods of silence are infrequent. Turn-taking occurs when comment or response flows from person to person. As participators we must adhere to the unspoken laws of timing: make our responses to someone's statement or question immediately or signal in some way a need for extra time, or the opportunity is lost as the conversation is taken over by someone else. Tom, like others with aphasia, cannot interpret and respond to information while remembering parts of what may have been said previously. Thus, the aphasic person's responses may be poorly timed, interruptive, or seemingly off the subject, or he may simply not respond at all. Unless others are aware of the problem and can make adjustments, they may unintentionally exclude the aphasic person. Consequently, aphasic persons may feel uncomfortable in group conversations, as Tom did, gaining little pleasure from the experience.

As the other spouses also reported, Lee misses the spontaneity of communicative flow. There is a constant need for her to slow down. When she feels excited about something and she wants to tell Tom, she must slow down first to avoid fragmented sentences, too much inflection, and too fast a delivery of her words.

Guidelines for Communicating

It is helpful to consider all these issues when communicating with those who have reduced auditory comprehension. Unfortunately, the aphasic individual is not able to make major adjustments; the burden of change is placed upon those around him. Since no two people are alike, a different combination of the problems we have described will be seen in each case, and the aphasic person's emotional reaction to these problems will likewise vary. It is important for recovery to respond to each person at a level best suited to him, preserving individuality. A speech and language pathologist should be consulted to learn exactly how the auditory system is involved. With treatment, and over time, auditory comprehension does improve, but it is impossible to predict exactly how much auditory function a person will recover: some comprehension changes may remain permanent. In speech and language treatment, exercises that focus on the problem areas will likely be recommended. Practicing these exercises provides stimulation, allowing the auditory skill to redevelop. At the same time, the learning of practiced compensatory strategies improves auditory functioning as well. There follows a list of those most commonly used by persons with aphasia and family members. As always, a speech and language pathologist should be consulted to determine which may be most useful in a particular case.

Suggestions for family members and others:

1. Establish auditory attention by saying the person's name or touching him before talking.
2. Maintain eye contact.
3. Allow the person "warm-up" time by casual social exchange before giving the most important part of your message.
4. Speak at a slightly slower rate: make pauses longer between sentences.
5. Keep the volume of your speech the same.
6. Avoid over-exaggerating the intonation of your voice.
7. Use the same vocabulary you always have used; avoid "talking down" to the person.
8. Think about your nonverbal communication, such as your facial expression, and keep it congruent with your verbal message.
9. Use gestures as you speak to point to and "act out" your message whenever possible.
10. Accompany your speech with visual information when possible, e.g., pictures and written words.
11. Provide contextual clues for the person who has difficulty associating the meaning of single words.
12. Repeat when it is requested or when important information is relayed.

13. Phrase information differently when repeating if the first message was unclear to the aphasic person.
14. Divide longer directions, comments, or questions into shorter sentences.
15. Allow the person extra time to absorb the message.
16. Avoid sudden conversational shifts.
17. Learn to recognize auditory overload, which signals time to take breaks.

Suggestions for persons with aphasia:

1. Concentrate on listening to the speaker's message, consciously tuning out distractions.
2. If you know you didn't understand, say so.
3. Ask questions about parts of the information to clarify.
4. When you are aware you are having problems understanding, ask the speaker:
   to repeat his message
   to say it a different way
   to show you what he means
   to write down his message.
5. Learn to read facial expressions; if you have responded in a conversation to the speaker's remark and his expression reflects puzzlement, ask if he is confused.
6. Tell fast speakers to slow down.
7. Ask others to stop for a moment when you need extra time to interpret what they have just said.
8. In noisy situations, excuse yourself for a few moments or go into a quieter room to help relieve overload.
9. If you fail to understand a conversation among a group, try drawing someone aside later and asking them to explain the discussion.
10. When you need a break, tell the speaker you will have to continue the conversation later.

Problems with Reading

Reading: for many it is a source of pleasure, an opportunity to gain knowledge, or a way to spend hours enjoying the beauty of the printed word. For others, reading may simply be a necessary activity for understanding advertisements, schedules, and other messages. No matter what the reading interest or need, most of us would find it devastating to be without this skill.

Aphasia changes reading ability. Some find it requires more concentration to read and remember narrative material, others may lose some recognition of the printed word. Occasionally an individual experiences a complete loss of word recognition, or alexia. Like the area of auditory comprehension just discussed, reading involves many different skills, so that reading difficulties are diverse.

Learning to read again following a stroke is not the same process as when we first acquired that skill. Adults have already developed proficiency, but the brain injury changes the ability to perform the different functions necessary to read easily. Retraining, then, first involves a careful analysis of what skills have been affected before exercises and strategies to improve the deficient areas can be practiced. Given time and work, reading can become functional again.

In this section we will look at the variety of reading problems after stroke and talk about recovery of that skill and compensations for the remaining deficits.

Visual Perception

Strokes, particularly those that occur in the posterior part of the left hemisphere of the brain, disrupt visual perception, the accurate assessment of what one sees. It is important to recognize that visual perception and visual acuity are *two separate skills.* (Visual acuity can also change after a stroke, with the patient suffering blurred or double vision. Physicians often recommend waiting a minimum of six months after the stroke before consulting an ophthalmologist or getting new glasses, since visual acuity can fluctuate a great deal at first.) When both visual acuity and visual perception are impaired, it can be difficult to assess the exact degree of each.

Although the two skills are so closely related, they are distinct. This analogy may explain the difference: suppose you see an apple on a table. If you have blurred vision, it will look fuzzy; with double vision you may see two apples; but in each case you recognize "apple." With visual perceptual problems, however, you may not perceive it as separate from the table; you may see only part of it; or you may note something red, not recognizing it as "apple."

To illustrate further, visual perception is what enables us to differentiate figures, as when we recognize that □ □ are two identical shapes, that △ ▽ are the same shapes but are inverted, that △ △ are different sizes, and that □ △ are two shapes but are not identical. We are also aware that ⟨∑⟩ is a whole but can be divided into two parts that fit together. Those who have problems seeing these differences in shapes and familiar objects also find seeing and remembering letters difficult, and they have particular trouble with such subtle changes as we see in the letters b, p, and d.

Many stroke survivors, such as Ed, can mistake visual perceptual problems as *changes* in vision. For months Ed complained that he just didn't know what was wrong with his glasses. He tried moving them up and down, tried doing without them entirely—all to no avail. He frequently asked for an appointment with an ophthalmologist and had a hard time understanding the need to wait. Because of his auditory comprehension problems, it took some time for him to realize his visual problems were perceptual in nature.

He did not always notice words and letters on one side of his visual field and had difficulty distinguishing similar letters. This was particularly traumatic for him, as his wife remembers: "Here was a man who used to scan the oatmeal box while eating breakfast and read an entire book in one hour, who now couldn't recognize the letters of the alphabet!" Today, although Ed has recovered his ability to recognize words and read books, he can do so for only brief periods of time and at a much slower rate than before.

Visual perceptual disturbances can easily cause persons to misread letters. Upper- and lowercase letters, cursive and printed styles, can be confused. Consider how the variety of print styles and sizes on variously colored backgrounds and kinds of paper changes the way written material looks, and you begin to see how a person with perceptual problems suffers. Larger print on good quality paper with well-spaced text is read most easily and is usually easiest for a stroke survivor to use first when reading once again.

Ted, like Ed, experienced both visual perceptual and acuity problems. To help, his ophthalmologist recommended using two pairs of glasses, reading glasses and his normal trifocals. Ted likes to use the large-print edition of the *Reader's Digest* when he reads longer material. Although he can read the newspaper, he finds the print seems to "run together," causing fatigue, overload, and thus limited endurance. Ted goes on to explain that many letters, like m, n, and h, are letters he sometimes reads backwards or upside down. As he tries to speed up his reading, he sees the wrong letters and can't figure out the word. This problem becomes more severe in longer words such as "condominium," where the syllables might be inverted and perceived as "conmindoium," a word that makes no sense to him.

Ted also has trouble differentiating similar words such as "conversion," "conversation," and "convention." He reads the words in the rest of the sentence to give himself a clue about context and thus, he hopes, meaning. If he is reading quickly and misperceives one of these similar-looking words, he may come to a faulty conclusion. Ted also cannot understand words divided with a hyphen at the end of a line since he does not see the word printed all together.

Treatment for these problems often involves developing concentration and attention to details of differences in letters. Ed practiced looking at both upper - and lowercase letters of varied size for quite some time during his rehabilitation program.

Decoding or Interpreting Word Meaning

Once a person has learned accurate perception and basic letter recognition, he must be able to decode, or get meaning from, letters and words. To accomplish this, a series of functions must take place in the brain. For example, to decode the word "complication," I must first recognize all the letters and remember the rules of dividing the word into syllables: "com pli ca tion." I then use phonetic pronunciation to figure out each syllable. When I get to the last syllable, "tion," I have to think of the phonetic irregularity that makes the "t" sound like "sh" when it is combined with "ion." After analyzing the units of the word, I put the parts together to make a meaningful word, "complication." Of course I am not aware of this process because my brain will perform these steps quickly and automatically.

We can see how complex this decoding process is if we look at our English alphabet. It includes nineteen consonants, five vowels, and the ambiguous letters y and w, all of which have names *and* sounds. In addition, c, g, and ch have both hard and soft sounds depending on the vowels following them. The vowels, a, e, i, o, and u, change their sounds depending on their position in a word, whether they are doubled, or whether they become a diphthong (ou, ow, oi, oy, ue, ew), as in cow and new. When consonants are put together to form consonant blends (bl, tr, str, etc.) or consonant digraphs (th, sh, ph, gh, ps, ck, kn, wh, wr), this adds even more complexity to the decoding process. Thus, there are many different sounds and combinations of sounds to remember.

When decoding is a problem, a person might look at a word, perhaps recognize all the letters, yet still be unable to make sense of it, or he may recognize words with "high visibility" like "table," "chair," and "apple," but still be unable to remember the sounds or names of the letters in them. When he sees a word he doesn't recognize, his brain, having lost an automatic decoding ability, has no strategy for figuring out what it is.

As Paula attempted reading again and had trouble remembering the letter names, she began tracing them on her leg, using her unaffected sense of touch to send a message to the brain. Persons with decoding problems also practice saying letter names, spelling a word out loud to help them decode. Ed found the most effective method for him was to copy the word on a piece of paper.

After a person learns to decode words by breaking them into separate letters and syllables, tachistoscopic training is sometimes used in treatment. In this training, words are flashed rapidly on a screen to help the brain "see" or synthesize the whole unit. According to current research, much of the normal process of reading involves this kind of recognition. Obviously, reading letter by letter is too laborious for any of us to read quickly. Our brains recognize familiar whole words without needing to do this type of analysis. We may find it necessary to break down words into letters and syllables when the term is unfamiliar, but not as a routine process. Tachistoscopic training, used as part of the rehabilitation program, can sometimes help speed up decoding to make reading more functional again.

Understanding Words, Sentences, and Paragraphs

Another ability needed to read "normally" is good reading comprehension, or skill in understanding words, sentences, and paragraphs. This is influenced by our vocabulary or word recognition, by the complexity of the grammar and syntax of our language, the length of the material, and our skill at putting everything together to understand the whole.

Ted described his experience to us: "Now when I read I feel like I'm in a room full of fog!" In this "fog," though he concentrated fully to interpret the meaning of the written material, he often still felt that complete understanding was beyond him.

A person with a reading problem has impaired ability to associate a written word with the meaning he has stored in his memory. Words (such as "table," "run," and "stop") that occur most frequently in the language and can easily be pictured, touched, or even smelled are easier to recognize. On the other hand, longer and more abstract words such as "adversary" or "architect" are less likely to be recognized. In a similar vein, nouns and verbs are easier than adjectives, adverbs, prepositions, and connective words. The more severe the aphasia, the more vocabulary recognition will be impaired.

It is important to remember that an aphasic person's ability to say the word out loud is *not* an indication of understanding. Ed often repeats a word when he is attempting to trigger recognition. Sometimes this technique is successful, sometimes not. When he is finally able to understand the word, this is often because he has "heard" himself, letting the auditory center of his brain recognize it when the visual center could not. Paula could not effectively use this technique since her verbal apraxia (see "Problems with Speaking" in Chapter 4) prevented her from fluently reading words out loud. It took so much concentration to remember how to say the word that by the time she could, meaning eluded her.

There are several strategies effective in gaining word meaning. It must be realized, however, that the success of any strategy is highly individual and dependent upon the extent of the brain injury. Further, it takes considerable time to explore and develop these techniques.

When we communicate, individual words are combined in a variety of ways to form sentences. Yet it is this variety that becomes confusing with aphasia. When we read, we are generally not consciously aware of sentence structure though at times varied sentences enhance our reading pleasure. But to the reader with aphasia, as sentences become longer and word order and grammar become more complicated, understanding suffers.

The easiest sentence for the aphasic person to understand is one containing only a subject, verb, and object, such as "The boy (subject) eats (verb) lunch (object)." A longer sentence with greater variety and complexity, such as "After the ballots had been counted, George, who was running for political office, asked for a recount" is more complicated to interpret. In this construction, the main sentence is "George asked for a recount." The subordinate clauses are added to tell when and why this event occurred and to give us more information about George. In a sentence like this, problems with comprehension occur because punctuation marks break the flow. In addition, the subject and the verb are separated and it is necessary to differentiate the main idea from less important ones. We see a similar example of complexity in: "If John is home tonight, you can come for dinner." An aphasic person may understand the main sentence, "you can come for dinner," but not the condition under which the event can occur.

The English language includes other sentence structures too numerous to delineate in this section. For those interested in the specific sentence constructions that are most difficult for those with aphasia, we have included an appendix, "Language Difficulties for the Aphasic Affecting Reading," for easy reference.

As we have just seen, then, word form (morphology) and word order (syntax) influence comprehension of what is read, but semantics, or interpretation of word meaning, can play a part as well. In this newspaper headline, "BUSH BOWS OUT OF THE RACE," each word might be interpreted several different ways. Ted enjoys scanning the sports section each day, but when he reads a caption such as "RANGERS DEEP-FREEZE THE TIGERS' BATS," that newspapers use to keep readers interested, he is really unsure as to who won the game. The headline may be exciting, but it is too abstract to give him any information. Furthermore, we use many idioms in our language that are frustrating to interpret for the aphasic reader. "Why are you so short with me?" is a sentence that may at face value appear to refer to size, not temperament. Many stroke survivors say they no longer enjoy choosing a humorous greeting card because they miss the point or find the attention-grabbing innuendo much too confusing.

In addition, groups of words with distinct but minute shades of meaning ("some," "none," "few") may be a problem since aphasic individuals understand the concept behind the words but confuse the exact degrees of meaning for each. Similarly, words that sound the same but are spelled differently (homonyms, e.g., "piece/peace" or "minor/miner") interfere with comprehension when the aphasic reader typically focuses on the one meaning that first pops into his mind, failing to realize that he needs to switch to another interpretation.

These examples illustrate how a reader with aphasia might get only part of the information he reads if he misses a change in a word, in word order, or in word meaning in a sentence. But most of our daily reading involves reading groups of sentences or paragraphs. Consider all the grammatical structures we have described thus far and envision trying to read an article in a newspaper. It now becomes easier to see why it is difficult for the aphasic person to get all the facts necessary to interpret the intent of the story.

Retention or Memory

Once written material is understood, we mentally store the most important information, using our skill of retention. To do this we continually filter relevant from irrelevant information automatically. None of us is able to recount everything from the morning paper by the end of the day, yet we are able to recall the main ideas and most important facts of articles having the greatest interest to us. Retention and memory abilities are also what enable us to pick up a book we are reading and resume at the correct page because we remember the information in the book thus far. This is not true of the aphasic reader; as Betty remarked, "If I read something in the evening, I can't . . . for the life of me remember what I have read by the time I get ready for bed!" With aphasia the brain loses the ability to hold the same amount of information over the same period of time as before. Betty can now retain more factual information but at first had no interest in reading as nothing stayed with her long enough to make it worthwhile. This happened in spite of her good word recognition and comprehension.

Aphasia reduces retention both during and after reading. If I am looking at a newspaper article and the information begins to exceed my capacity to remember it, by the end of the article I won't be able to put all the facts together to get an appropriate impression because I have not remembered all of them along the way. Rereading, increasing concentration, frequently pausing, and repeating out loud are often helpful—but this is time-consuming and fatiguing. Those who have mastered decoding and comprehension find that better retention of written material comes only with persistence. Many suggest that setting aside a certain time each day to read helps force them to practice consistently.

Drawing Inferences and Forming Conclusions

Another area for discussion is our ability to draw inferences and form conclusions from what we are reading. We have already mentioned how the difficulties of understanding word form, order, or meaning along with faulty retention disrupt the ability to get all the facts accurately. But a reader must also reason, analyze, draw inferences, and form conclusions. To do this, one must have intact thought organization and memory. With reduced rate of reading and faulty retention these assumed abilities may be compromised. Therefore the aphasic might get "hooked" on one thought while reading, and form erroneous inferences and conclusions based on limited or faulty retention of the facts. Treatment for those with difficulties in thought organization can involve extracting information systematically either by writing down the main points or dictating them into a tape recorder. Using this method, the aphasic person can then, after several reviews of the material, draw inferences and conclusions, one idea at a time. This is time-consuming but, according to stroke survivors, a necessary process to assimilate and integrate complex information accurately.

Functional Reading

Understanding advertisements, menus, schedules, theater listings, telephone directories, etc., is another important facet of reading. It is necessary for those with aphasia to slowly and methodically scan all the information. Since these materials are not typically organized systematically, the chance of missing relevant facts is increased. To help, stroke survivors say they need to divide this material into smaller sections, often using a handheld guide to isolate each part.

In reading an advertisement, for instance, we are first drawn to the most visible information, most likely written in the largest print. Next, we can read the information in smaller print to find details like place, time, date, etc., noting exclusions or conditions put in hard-to-see places. Those with limited reading and retention find this more of a chore and often fail to notice information in fine print. Then, too, ads that rely on fewer words to attract attention can be easily misunderstood.

Menus have varied formats, often not only listing foods but including elaborate descriptions. The more varied this visual presentation is, the more difficult reading it will be. In addition, pressure to order rapidly from the menu can cause added stress. (Those who frequent the same restaurant might take a menu home and become familiar with it before the next visit.)

Schedules of any type present similar problems in that reviewing to assure all information has been read, understood, and incorporated into memory is time-consuming. Information may be presented under various headings and contain exclusions that must be noted before making an informed decision. The exclusions in travel schedules often seem to be in the smallest print or even on another page, intentionally placed in hopes readers will miss them. Practice without time pressure in a "safe" environment and the use of compensatory strategies seem to be the most effective ways to relearn how to handle these important materials.

Conclusion

Accurate reading demands that many abilities be intact. Problems in just one area may be so defeating to an individual that he loses further interest in reading. Although Tom now reads the daily newspaper, it is so difficult and slow that he doesn't really enjoy it. Still, his gradual improvement is enough to keep him motivated. Paula, who has recently started reading books again, can only go through a few pages before her problems with retention start to interfere. It frustrates her that she cannot pick up the book the next day and resume reading without painstaking review. Both Tom and Paula find reading retention still fluctuates daily and reading speed is, and always will be, reduced considerably. Ted has found the process of decoding so laborious it prevents him from reading as he used to. He no longer can rely on it as a source of relaxation and a way to keep informed about the world. A good substitute for him has been Talking Books, a federally funded program available free of charge through local libraries. As part of this program, books and magazines are taped for people with reading difficulties and sent upon request to their homes. (See appendix, "Reading Materials for the Reader with Aphasia," for more information about this service.)

Because we have made the assumption that people need some degree of reading ability to function well in our society, we feel it is important to discover where breakdown with aphasia occurs and how best to work with each problem. Although it takes time to read again following a stroke, a speech and language pathologist trained in diagnosing and remediating problems can help. Some of the more common compensatory strategies often suggested in a treatment program are:

1. Reduce reading rate.
2. Trace or orally spell to assist in decoding unfamiliar words.
3. Develop an outline of what information you might expect to find in the material *before* you read it.
4. Read out loud when speech problems do not interfere.
5. Pause frequently to think about the content of what you have just read.
6. Use a guide or your finger to track the line you are reading to limit your visual field.
7. Reread confusing sentences.
8. Underline key words.
9. Outline what you have read, using key words and phrases to help recall.
10. When speech skills allow, discuss what you have read with someone else.

Regular practice in reading for the aphasic person is essential.

Problems with Speaking

Our ability to speak enables us to connect with one another in a dimension unequaled elsewhere in the animal kingdom. While communication does occur without speech as we move, gesture, and use facial expression, speech represents the most sensitive and elaborate form of communication that exists. It allows us the freedom to instruct, describe, entertain, command, reveal feelings and opinions, and ask questions. Aphasia can strip an individual of this ability, leaving him fully aware of what is going on around him but without an avenue to express his needs, thoughts, and ideas. We listen to our voice and recognize its unique tone, pitch, and rhythm; with expressive speech and language problems, speech often sounds so different that it seems almost as if a stranger is now residing within. Many different speech and language patterns can result from aphasia, depending on the area of the brain injured. Tom, Ed, Paula, Betty, Ted, and Carl shared their thoughts and reactions of managing through a time when communicating verbally seemed almost impossible.

Normally, we are not conscious of our speech. But as we talk, our brains automatically access several speech and language systems concurrently. To produce coherent speech, competence is required in the areas of phonology (sound production), syntax (word order), morphology (word forms), semantics (word meaning), and pragmatics (nonverbal messages). As a child first learns to communicate he uses single words, often accompanied by a gesture. Next, he combines two words that may communicate an action, a location, a description, or show possession. For instance, he may say such things as, "Go store," "mommy talk," or "baby toy." As speech develops, the sounds of the language, or phonology, become refined, starting with those most easily produced and progressing to more involved sound combinations. The first spoken words are those that express complete meaning and are most frequently used in a language; less frequently occurring and longer words demand the ability to sequence sounds and syllables and are acquired later. As speech develops to the two-word level and beyond, consideration must then be given to the arrangement of words in an utterance, the syntax. In addition, language development requires a knowledge of the morphology of that language, or the understanding that one word can take several forms. For example, other forms of the verb "go" are "went," or "gone"; the noun "baby" could take the form "babies" or "baby's." As speech and language becomes complex, more thought is given to the exact meaning of words, or semantics. A knowledge of semantics insures we have said what we really intended (e.g., "devastating," "awful," "unpleasant," as opposed to "bad"). Finally, we learn to refine the pragmatics of conversational interchange, becoming able to change the tone and inflection of our voice and the context in which the information is given to indicate the intent of our messages.

With aphasia, competence in one or more of these essential speech and language areas breaks down. It is important to note that remediating expressive speech and language problems, as we discussed with regard to reading, will not be the same as learning a language for the first time. Even though persons with aphasia may have lost their ability to communicate verbally, they were once able to talk quite well.

An important distinction to make is that all speech problems of those with aphasia do not sound the same. In some, speaking attempts may produce limited or no sound. In others, enough words to express immediate needs may be possible but more complex communication is nonexistent. Still other persons might verbalize continuous strings of words and phrases that convey little meaning or even nonsense. The literature about strokes and aphasia suggests that injury in the anterior portion of the brain's left hemisphere makes speech sound telegraphic—that is, there are nouns and verbs but no "filler" words. With this type of problem one might hear, "He go store" or simply, "store." This is sometimes referred to as Broca's aphasia, named for the physician who first wrote about the disorder. By contrast, involvement in the posterior portion of the brain produces a fluent speech wherein a person can talk in complete sentences but uses words that express little or no meaning. This is sometimes called Wernicke's aphasia, again named for the person who first described the syndrome. With this problem one might hear, "I go see around flourt over there before me." (While one should be familiar with these terms, it will be most helpful for our purposes to consider only the characteristics of aphasic speech and language disorders.)

A question that often arises when addressing problems with verbal communication is the distinction between "speech" and "language." Language encompasses the areas of word form, word order, word meaning, and the context in which these words are uttered. Speech, on the other hand, refers to how we form and produce the sounds needed to talk. First we will focus on problems occurring after stroke that affect only speech.

Dysarthric Speech

Dysarthric speech results when there is weakness in some or all of the structures we use when we talk. These include our larynx (voice box), pharynx (throat), tongue, and lips. When any of these structures become weakened following an injury to the brain, the way we sound changes. Problems with respiration occur when muscles that contract to force air through the vocal cords are weak. Resonance (vibration) will be reduced if the pharyngeal muscles are weak, and articulation is affected if the tongue, lips, and facial muscles are involved. The weakness will occur on the side of the body that is contralateral (opposite) to the site of the brain injury, sometimes producing a noticeable drooping of the mouth. (The weakness in the larynx and the pharynx may be pronounced enough to cause problems with chewing and swallowing as well.) Dysarthric speech that affects articulation is easily recognized as similar to that of someone who is intoxicated, as it is slurred, distorted, and imprecise. The weakness reduces the speed or rate of talking, the strength of tongue and lip movement, and the articulation or precision with which individual sounds can be produced. There are several types of dysarthric speech, depending on the area of the brain affected, although we will not elaborate here. Suffice it to say that techniques to overcome dysarthria often involve conscious slowing of the rate of speech and relearning where to place the lips and tongue in the absence of any kinesthetic feedback. The effect of speaking with dysarthria is similar to trying to talk after an injection of novocaine.)

Verbal Apraxia

A second speech problem is verbal apraxia. This difficulty results in errors in speech production different from dysarthria in that paralysis is not responsible for the problem. Whereas dysarthric speech is filled with distortions of sounds, apraxic speech has more substitutions and additions of sounds and syllables. In dysarthria, the word "refrigerator" may be produced as "re fhri sh er a der," and in apraxia may be pronounced as "re for ger a shion." When a person has verbal apraxia, the brain no longer sends accurate information on how to position the speech mechanisms to form sounds and words. This can happen either in the larynx, causing an individual to actually have trouble starting a sound, or in the articulators, so that the ability to position the tongue, lips, and teeth to talk is impaired. As the combinations of sounds get more complex (e.g., "thermostat" versus "bed"), such errors become more apparent. It should be pointed out that apraxia can occur without an expressive aphasia (changes in how a person talks because he can't think of words or how to put them together in sentences). If apraxia is severe enough so that no speech can be produced, it will mask the extent of the underlying language involvement. Only as the speech finally emerges can the extent of the language difficulty be determined. While a person who is apraxic may produce sound inadvertently—such as a moan in pain or a word as he attempts to gesture—he does not have *volun-*

tary control over sound and speech production. Tom, who had a severe apraxia, could "hear" the sound in his head but nothing seemed to work together when he went to say it.

While there are numerous ways to treat apraxia of speech, all basically involve creating awareness of how voluntary sound is finally produced, harnessing this awareness, and using it to "re-program" the brain to make purposeful sounds and words. Persons with verbal apraxia may still be able to say certain words because they come so automatically they don't need this sound programming; examples are swear words, greetings, and sometimes a few names or nouns. Sometimes activities that trigger recall of a familiar series (e.g., counting, saying the days of the week, or singing "Happy Birthday") may be helpful to stimulate production of words again.

As speech began to return for Carl, he became frustrated that he could not produce certain words consistently after much practice. Since this is very common with apraxia, the individual needs reassurance that he is not regressing. Carl also experienced perseveration. His brain became so overloaded or taxed that he repeated the same word or phrase continuously. Here again, reassurance needs to be given that this happens with recovery, and the patient must be reminded that to say what he wants he needs to rest before trying the desired word again. When speech problems are severe, a perseverated word might be the only thing a person can express, and no amount of rest will break his pattern. Other strategies our families used to produce a word included writing the first letter of it, drawing pictures, and gesturing. To demonstrate how effective and creative this kind of strategy can be: one person with severe apraxia, unable to say the word "Toyota," gestured it instead by slanting his eyes with his fingers. If the listener thinks he knows the intended word, he might help by saying a leading sentence like, "I eat my soup with a ——," enabling the individual to say "spoon."

Tom, Carl, and Paula all have verbal apraxia. None of them had any ability to voluntarily produce sound immediately following the stroke. As Tom struggled with his apraxia and aphasia, he felt like a baby learning the language for the first time. He first had to learn to make individual sounds again, sounds that would later become words. Next he practiced combining these words into simple sentences. Yet speech emerged only with maximum effort. He would "grab hold of" certain phrases and expressions that were easy to produce and repeat them continually. His family

remembers him repeating "That's the key" in most communicative attempts. Tom's voice also sounded different to him,
rather slow and labored and without its usual pitch and inflection.

Carl's apraxia continues to prevent him from initiating very
many words. He communicates primarily through single words
accompanied by gestures and pantomine, much like charades,
often giving himself and his listener other cues by writing the
first letter of the word or drawing pictures on paper or in the air—
all of which help him to say the word or communicate an idea.

Paula notes that her speech still fluctuates daily and is influenced by fatigue and stress. She has also remarked, as have other
women, that her speech is worse during her period. At first Paula
had trouble initiating speech, a common problem with apraxia in
that the larynx almost needs a "push" to get started. As she improved, she became more able to start a word but then had trouble
sequencing the sounds in it. Attempting to say "potato," for instance, she might instead say "topato." Paula could not hear what
she was saying; the words were often unintelligible and she didn't
sound like herself. Both dyspraxia and dysarthria cause tone,
pitch, and rhythm to alter. Paula's speech is now slow and labored; she still rehearses what to say and thinks how best to say
it. Recalling her days as a supervisor of sales representatives,
when her well-articulated speech was her trademark, she still has
trouble reconciling how difficult it is for her to say words and
formulate her thoughts.

Language-Based Difficulties

How then do deficiencies in language areas affect verbal expression? The aphasic individual must first think what he wants
to say. Next, he must find the words to communicate this message and put those words in the proper order (syntax) and the right
form (morphology). If, for instance, an aphasic person wanted to
say, "The lady in the red dress who lives across the street from me
had been crying because her puppy was run over by a car," he
might only be able to get out, "Girl . . . sad . . . puppy . . . car."
When Tom tried to convey a long message like this, he could only
produce the essential words to communicate the most critical
part of his message, which sounded somewhat like a telegram.
The rest was just too long and involved to recall, put in sequential
order, and relay. After hearing his reduced messages, his wife

often had to ask questions to get more details. Tom *knew* what he intended to say and had some of the words, but he couldn't organize them in his head to express them. Lee's questions helped him focus on one part of his message and say a word, use a gesture, or draw a picture to get out the ideas piece by piece. His original thought was often finally expressed, but in an extremely painstaking and often disorganized way.

At times Lee wondered why Tom's words came out all "scrambled." She came to learn that as the aphasic person strives to communicate, the message is given priority over the form. It is too difficult to incorporate the rules of grammar to change the form of the word depending on its location and use in the sentence. For example, pronouns may be used incorrectly when a person with aphasia is aware that one is needed but can't recall which to use. Thus, "My father, he . . . " may be expressed as "My father, she . . . ".

With such syntactic and morphological problems, speech can be reduced to a very simple level. While some complex sentences may be heard occasionally, the aphasic individual's messages are shorter and less detailed than they were before his stroke. It also takes a lot more time to say even these short messages. Tom remarked at one point that friends thought he "sounded better now," but he was well aware how hard he always had to concentrate on word usage, word form, and sentence organization as he conversed. His speech lacked variety and was less complete than it was before his stroke. When he is engaged in a conversation, his speech is formulated so slowly that he has trouble talking with more than one person at a time and feels he is always "one step behind"; by the time he organizes what he wants to say and thinks about how to say it, everyone else is on to the next topic.

Eventually Tom began to realize that speaking was only one part of resuming communication. To converse effectively he had to listen to another person, assign meaning to what he heard, and then organize his own thoughts before he could formulate and combine words to reply. He remembers the first time he told a joke. As he tried to keep the punch line in mind he kept confusing the order of events in the story. Without his former rapid delivery of speech, his audience got lost as to the sequence of events. When the punch line came, no one, including Tom, knew how he had gotten there! Everything that had once happened automatically was now a time-consuming and exhausting process.

We have talked about language problems resulting from disruptions in the ability to order words in messages and use appropriate grammar. Those who experience a stroke with injury to the posterior portion of the brain, as we mentioned, have an expressive language difficulty characterized by speech that is full of words but lacking in content. In the example, "The table flew to the right of the chair," the sentence is grammatically correct but the meaning is erroneous. This statement may sound fine to the aphasic whose difficulty involves problems with semantics. An expressive language problem of this type can be quite confusing to the uninformed listener, since the aphasic's speech has the proper rhythm, tone, and pitch. The listener may suddenly find himself feeling he has missed something. It can be equally devastating to the aphasic individual, who may not really "hear" what he's said.

Ed spoke copiously after his stroke without realizing he was conveying little information. Unless the listener signaled or stopped him, he would skip from sentence to sentence repeatedly. He assumed he had made his point unless he was faced with a confused look or an incorrect response to his comment. The first sign that a fluent aphasic is recovering is his ability to once again "listen" to what he is saying. He may not be able to correct his errors yet, but at least he is more cognizant of his mistakes. As Ed improved, he learned to watch others' expressions, pausing to check his communications for redundancy and clarity by asking, "What did I just say?"

Ted had always been a talker. In spite of his aphasia he still had lots to say but never remembered if he had said it before. While his initial conversations were fraught with repetition, he is now able to listen to himself more easily and to watch others' responses to check his communication.

People with a fluent aphasia may use what are called literal and verbal paraphasias. A literal paraphasia is usually a sound substitution in a word; it may be an end sound that emerges both at the beginning and ending of a word, as in, "lencil" for "pencil." Some of these jargon words are hard to associate with the intended word. If, for instance, the word "flourt" was substituted for flower, it might only be understood in the context of the rest of the statement. A verbal paraphasia, on the other hand, is a substitution of an entire real word. If the word is related (e.g., "table" for "chair"), it is easier to interpret than unrelated substitutions such as "pretty" for "flower." These paraphasias can sometimes sound similar to the speech of an individual with apraxia, causing confusion about the nature of the disorder: is it a speech or language problem? It is important to remember that a speech and language pathologist will treat the problem and not the label, with the goal of facilitating as much return of one's expressive abilities as possible.

Dysnomia

One expressive language disorder, anomia or dysnomia, refers to difficulty in naming objects or in retrieving the desired word and "having what you want to say on the tip of your tongue." It happens to all of us on occasion, particularly as we age, but becomes more frequent with aphasia. Circumlocution, or the process of skirting the desired word and replacing it with similar words, is a strategy most often used by people with this problem. Many become so adept at this that the listener is quite unaware that another word has been substituted. One individual, struck by the number of words in our language with closely related meanings, would visualize a television screen listing similar words to help him find the right one. He would become frustrated when, as so often happened, the chosen word was "just off" in meaning from the word he really wanted. Frequently he would find himself using even more complex words than he normally would have in an attempt to get closer to the one he really wanted.

Since the proper names of people and places are highly specialized words, difficulty in retrieving them is one of the most commonly experienced language problems in aphasia and seems to be one of the last skills to return with recovery. This problem creates untold frustration, especially to those who pride themselves on name recall and may have used this skill readily at work and in social situations. Many can successfully use strategies of association to help access the names they want. For instance, a street with the name "Maple" could be associated with a tree, or a person named "Bill" might be paired with a gesture indicating money.

Ted continues to have a severe dysnomia. His best strategy at first was to compile a small notebook of words he frequently needed to say. Since he was able to read them, he would look in his notebook whenever he couldn't retrieve a word. He also chose certain words to memorize and repeat out loud until they were incorporated into his vocabulary. While running with his dog, for example, he was constantly asked the name of the breed.

Frustrated over his inability to retrieve and say "Airedale," he wrote it in his notebook and practiced repeating it as he ran. Needless to say, he was most excited when someone *finally* asked him the question and he could immediately reply, "Airedale!" That person could never have realized what a struggle it had been for Ted to get to that point.

Ted also uses circumlocution as he talks. When he is unable to produce a similar word, he has learned to be very creative in his descriptions: "running shorts" become "small pants," his cardiologist is "the heart doctor," his surgical suit is called "greens," and the rehabilitation specialists are "the stroke people." The primary factor in Ted's inability to return to his job of selling computer supplies and pharmaceuticals was the severity of his dysnomia. He now sells electrical services in a position where he can effectively rehearse what he wants to say and sell the product but does not have to remember highly technical and complex names. Ted still has trouble listening to what he says as he gives a sales pitch, so he relies on looking at his listener's eyes to see if he has communicated his idea clearly. He becomes particularly annoyed when he orders from a menu and, thinking he has placed the order correctly, ends up with the wrong food. As Ted says, "That's when you learn how important it is to laugh at yourself."

Pragmatics

Our vocabulary, grammar, and the articulation of our speech combine to form the context of a verbal message, but there is far more to sending a verbal message than words alone. As Tom mentioned, once he learned to speak again, he had to relearn "the art of conversation." Pragmatics includes knowing when we should take turns in a conversation and the purpose of the communication. Is it, for instance, to inform, excite, or persuade? As we speak, we constantly change our body postures, facial expression, eye contact, and the tone and inflection of our voice to cue our listeners as to the real meaning behind the exchange. Making such adjustments involves a quick assessment of the social context of the situation where the conversation is taking place. Adjustments are also made according to how familiar we are with those involved as well as whether the exchange occurs at work or at leisure. We also consider our previous knowledge of our listener and the kind of interchange this person or group responds to best.

For example, should we be concerned with presenting only the facts or is some elaboration needed? Would it be appropriate to tell a joke? How familiar is our listener with the subject under discussion? To engage in conversation at this language level the speaker must be aware of the others' perspective. Persons with aphasia lose ability to assess the situation and integrate these factors, particularly at the speed at which conversational exchanges normally occur. Their concentration and energies are directed at just getting the content of the message accurate, leaving little resources remaining to focus on the pragmatics of the exchange.

The resulting impression may be that the aphasic individual is "slightly off" in his manner of communication. His timing in interjecting comments may be too late, since it has taken him much longer to form the words to express an idea. His shift to a new topic may be premature. Once he has succeeded in completing an idea in his head, he goes ahead and says it before the thought fades, unaware of the current focus of conversation. Tom's response to a question involves elaborating on everything he can remember about the subject, at times making him forget the original thought. Unless someone is able to "pull him back" to make his point, he can go on far too long, violating the unspoken rules of turn-taking we use constantly in conversation. The aphasic person's repertoire of speech acts is reduced so that he no longer persuades, questions, or informs, but simply responds when addressed. He may appear to monopolize the conversation because his expression takes longer. He may talk from one idea to the next without stopping for feedback or turn-taking in the conversation. He does not initiate speech, partly because his repertoire of social phrases is not readily available in his memory. Finally, the aphasic person is unable to use nonverbal signals of differing facial expressions and body posturing to add refinement or innuendo to his exchanges because he must concentrate so hard on what he is saying. A switch in focus to try to maintain eye contact, for example, would cause him to lose the thought.

Ted adds that with so much of his time spent coping with his aphasia and because it takes so much longer to get new information either by hearing it or reading it, his supply of subject matter for conversations is limited. He finds this to be an area he constantly strives to improve so he can be a more active participant in exchanges with others, but as "everything else with stroke, this, too, is *hard!*"

Cognition

It is worth repeating that although aphasia reduces a person's ability to verbally express his thoughts, it *does not* impair the existence of those thoughts. Intelligence is not compromised. Cognition, or our ability to perceive our world and classify information, is preserved. Rather, the speed in which the brain can process information coming in and formulate messages to send out is slower. Some with aphasia say this makes them feel intellectually deficient—as if they were on a slow train watching the rest of the world speed by. Tom remembers one occasion when he felt a tremendous pain in his side, was aware it needed to be checked, and attempted to communicate his thoughts to a nurse but was unable to express the idea completely. Thinking he was constipated, the nurse gave him an enema. In another instance, Tom emphatically responded, "No!" when his wife asked him if he wanted his watch set, in spite of his real intent to say "Yes." One can easily see how those interacting with the aphasic individual could falsely assume he is confused, unaware, and perhaps even mentally deficient.

Aphasia can also be misinterpreted as a behavioral problem, as in Paula's case. While she was sitting in her backyard one afternoon, a neighbor approached and greeted her. When Paula tried to say "Hi," she loudly proclaimed "Shit!" instead. Needless to say, the neighbor did not stop to talk. Many spouses report concerns that their husbands or wives no longer call them by family or pet names. They are puzzled as to how the aphasic person could have "lost" their identity. They may try to teach this lost name, but need to remember it is the speech difficulty masking recall.

With stroke recovery, speech and language competence will improve, yet deficiencies in organizing thoughts on as complete and complex a level as desired remain. As an aphasic person attempts to explain his thoughts and ideas, these may seem limited and inflexible. For example, imagine that an aphasic person needs to be included in his family's decision to buy a new car. The first step in making this decision is to think about the information available about the different cars. Next one needs to access one's long-term memory to determine what one already knows about buying cars. With aphasia, the process of pulling out this stored information, classifying and organizing it, and then screening out relevant from irrelevant data is disrupted. The aphasic person has trouble holding several thoughts in his head long enough to shift them around to consider the importance of each. He may "get stuck" thinking about only one of these factors because memory of the others has faded. Even though one fact may not be the most important one, it becomes the one he is able to discuss because it has stayed in his memory. So while the rest of the family is considering the car's fuel economy, he might be focused on the color of the upholstery. His approach to evaluating the car could be viewed by his family as limited or irrelevant. They may assume he lacks good judgment because he seems to think the upholstery color is more relevant than fuel economy. They may think he is drifting off on a tangent without seeing the point. Instead, this is really a reflection of his internal problems in retrieving, organizing, and storing all the information about the subject at one time, not an indication that he has lost his mental agility and is unable to have rational thoughts when it comes to purchasing a car.

Experiences of Stroke Survivors and Their Families

Although aphasia affects all areas of communication, the most observable one is verbal expression. Spouses and family members of our six stroke survivors remember all too clearly how frightening it was to be cut off from communication with their family member. At the onset of the stroke, these stroke survivors found themselves unaware of the magnitude of communication loss. Many remember discovering while hospitalized that they were unable to talk; interestingly, most were not frightened but were angry and frustrated over their failed attempts to talk.

Lee felt devastated by Tom's inability to communicate since he was "her best friend," the person to whom she turned daily to discuss her thoughts and concerns. To lose this important connection was almost too much to bear. It has taken time to reestablish communication, and many of their exchanges are still difficult. There is no longer the easy give and take of previous years, and she now has to plan times to communicate, knowing it will take longer and perhaps lead to frustration. She remembers one incident in particular during Tom's struggle to become his own communicator once again. One night while they enjoyed some needed time together at a restaurant, he was finally able to order from the menu without asking her for assistance. An event we handle with ease and relatively little thought was a monumental achievement for him.

Julie and Alice both miss the communication that always flowed so easily with their spouses. To Julie it seemed that her husband always tried harder when he talked to others. It may help to remember that a person with aphasia always has to be "on" to talk. While those without aphasia can be thinking of other things yet respond almost automatically without spending a great deal of time planning and organizing a reply, this is impossible for the aphasic. Aphasic persons may speak less at home because they are exhausted from communicating all day; now they see home as a place to recharge their batteries. Alice misses spontaneity when she's with her husband. It is most apparent during those times when she is having a bad day or dealing with a multitude of pressing problems. She knows Ted needs to communicate for himself but she loses the patience to wait for him to finish his thoughts on these days. The reality of living with someone with a speech problem is that it is easier sometimes than at others. The family member has his good and bad days just as the stroke survivor does. It is hard to be constantly reminded of the loss of an important part of any relationship: sharing through verbal exchange.

Suggestions

The following thoughts and ideas may help those living or interacting with stroke survivors. Remember that formulation of speech is slower and, therefore, extra time has to be allowed for the aphasic person to talk. This is most apparent in an exchange involving more than one individual. When someone is struggling to communicate and you think you know what he is trying to say, it is hard to decide when and if you should rescue him. Most people with aphasia agree that they prefer to signal for help in some way when they need it. Avoid finishing sentences for the aphasic person and ask leading questions that focus on his intended message instead. If you have a general idea of the subject, offer choices and then wait while he reiterates.

At first many aphasics panic when the desired message does not come. Learning to work through these communication blocks on their own, they say, makes it easier the next time. It may be helpful to discuss with the stroke survivor how he would like to manage this before it happens. Since, as we will discuss in the chapter "Psychosocial Issues Related to Stroke and Aphasia," self-esteem is a problem for those who have difficulty with communication, letting the stroke survivor resolve the communication difficulty by himself will enhance his feeling of self-worth.

Another question often voiced is whether to correct the aphasic person when he makes a statement that is either erroneous or grammatically incorrect. There is no right answer to this, only a need to exercise your judgment as to what is best for all involved. If you choose not to correct at the time, it might be agreeable to tell him later. Alice remembers that Ted was always confusing "yesterday," "today," and "tomorrow." Now that he has more self-confidence and understands aphasia better, she will at times correct him. At the beginning, this would have only frustrated him as he was unable to remember the correction to use appropriately the next time.

It is a good idea to allow the aphasic individual to do as much communicating for himself as possible, making note of progress with recovery. Certain communicative responsibilities the spouse may have handled at first can eventually be returned to the stroke survivor as he becomes ready. This will enhance further development of his communication and help him feel more "like his old self."

Betty reacted to the telephone initially with terror. Often she would slam down the receiver because she couldn't say what she wanted. Now she uses the phone with regularity, but it took time to overcome her fright. Tom was afraid his speech would not come quickly so he avoided answering the phone or making calls for a long time, not wanting to make a fool of himself. Using the phone is more difficult than face-to-face communication because the aphasic person can't use important clues by observing facial expressions of his listener. Daily experiences such as making appointments, asking for tickets at a theater, and finding items in a store are much easier to let someone else handle. But with practice and rehearsal, an individual with communication loss can develop strategies to handle his daily communicative needs. Before speaking on the phone, for instance, he can rehearse what he wants to say with a familiar, and therefore less threatening, individual. By doing this, the person with language difficulty can accustom himself to the pauses that seem to occur as he uses the phone. Knowing he can handle a situation alone is important to his emerging self-confidence.

Ted notes that it is stressful to speak when he is in a new and unanticipated situation. When he first started driving again he was involved in a minor car accident. Tom was understandably shaken; his limited speech added to his uncertainty. Nonetheless, he was able to handle the problem and so gained confidence. Many who know they will face a situation in which they are under pressure to talk find that speaking into a tape recorder or jotting down important information helps them to rehearse and prepare.

Finally, people with aphasia stress, "Don't pretend to understand." Those with speech difficulty are normally aware by the listener's facial expression when they have not relayed the appropriate message. Pretending comprehension reinforces the aphasic person's feelings that his communications are not valued and robs him of an opportunity to try again. While formal speech and language treatment forces aphasics to practice, they need to know they can talk outside the structure of their treatment sessions. The more they are allowed to practice and get positive feedback, the better the opportunity for improvement.

Problems with Writing

For want of a nail the shoe was lost
For want of a shoe the horse was lost
For want of the horse the battle was lost
For want of the battle the war was lost . . .

Writing is a complex expressive act requiring that several language systems be intact to perform many steps. When we write from our imagination, we must first generate and organize an idea, retrieve the necessary vocabulary to express it, formulate this thought into grammatically appropriate sentence form, encode word sounds into written letter symbols, transmit this final product into a motor act, and then execute this act by moving the pen or pencil with our hand over paper. This is fine when systems are operating efficiently, but interrupt this balanced chain at any point and the entire process becomes compromised. We have already discussed the ways aphasia reduces such capabilities as vocabulary retrieval, thought organization, and grammatical efficiency; we will now examine some of the ways expressing an idea in writing may be disrupted by aphasia and consider strategies to compensate for those difficulties.

Motor Skills

It is important to understand that because of its complexity, writing is nearly always impaired in aphasia, especially when verbal expression is also affected. Furthermore, it can often be the most noticeable problem in mild cases of aphasia. Writing skills may be among the last to redevelop following stroke and can remain impaired permanently to some degree. (To reiterate a point we have emphasized throughout this book, each person's aphasia is different, and the extent of the writing problem will vary. Emotional reactions to a writing problem also vary from one person to another.) It can be frightening for the stroke survivor to try to write for the first time only to discover he can't even sign his name, which may often happen early in his hospital stay before he has had much opportunity to learn about the difficulties caused by the aphasia. Much support and encouragement is useful at this time so that it is understood that practice can result in improvement. Betty, Ted, Paula, Tom, Carl, and Ed all were disturbed by their loss of writing ability. They challenged themselves to tackle this disability and have found indeed that they were able to make progress.

When we examine the process of writing more closely, we must consider the effects of paralysis or weakness of the affected hand. Betty, Tom, Paula, and Carl all lost use of their preferred (right) hand after the stroke and were faced with the task of learning to hold and guide a pen with their left hand. Paula was upset by the meaningless scribbling she made initially. All stressed how slowly proficiency with their left hand developed, in some cases taking several months. Most learned proper grip and paper placement first. Next they practiced copying large shapes and letters, then printing smaller letters, and eventually they learned cursive script again. Tom believes nothing short of constant daily practice with such drills led to his eventual success; it helped him to develop the fine motor skills necessary for gripping and moving the pen and forming each letter. In cases of partial paralysis a stroke survivor may first compensate by learning to write with the nonpreferred hand until enough strength and motor control has redeveloped to allow use of the dominant hand again. Some persons find that even after they are once again able to use their preferred hand, their writing now looks different due to hand weakness and thus different letter formation. Writing more slowly and stopping more frequently can be effective in improving writing legibility.

A second factor sometimes affecting motoric execution of writing is limb apraxia. An analogy will be helpful in understanding this confusing disorder. Imagine yourself in the middle of a nightmare in which you are being chased but can't move. Most of us have had such dreams where we can't run away even though we try. We aren't paralyzed but the urgent message to run just isn't making the legs and feet move. This is a simplified explanation of limb apraxia. Persons having it are unable to efficiently initiate and control voluntary movements with their hands or body. This disorder is usually associated with damage in the anterior portions of the brain and can affect gestural ability, the ability to use objects appropriately, and the ability to write. It is important to realize this is not because of paralysis to the arm, although some persons may also have muscular weakness. Limb apraxia affects only volitional (voluntary) movement because the message sent from the brain never makes it to the arm, leg, etc., or, if it does make it, is transmitted erroneously. The individual may not be able to initiate the act of writing when he is holding a pencil or may not be able to accurately complete words or sentences on paper. As with verbal apraxia, a person may make these same movements on an *in*voluntary basis. Again, drills with copying and initiating writing are often helpful in improving this condition.

Problems and Strategies

Aphasic impairment also changes the content of written material. Spelling very often becomes more difficult and less accurate. This occurs when the part of the brain responsible for encoding (retrieving the correct letter or letters to match the phonological sounds in our language) is damaged, and can range from total inability to spell to occasional letter deletions, additions, or substitutions. Three years after Carl's stroke, he finds he can just now begin to generate the first letter or two of an intended word. Betty remembers how dismayed she felt when she realized her spelling was awful. Not only was it impossible to recall how to spell words, she could not remember how to form individual letters either. A previously good speller, she felt like a child again. Although Betty was aware of her misspellings, many persons with aphasia are not. They may write a word that does not even look like the intended one yet believe it is correct. This is because the brain centers responsible for recognizing mistakes are also damaged. In fact, increasing this awareness in rehabilitation is a critical step in recovery. The person with aphasia may rely upon the feedback of others to tell him whether the word is correct until he learns to see his own mistakes and how to change them. For some time Ted wrote his lunch order as "tuna and cock," misspelling the word "coke" without realizing it. Doubtless this led to some interesting reactions, but with practice he was able to fix the mistake.

During treatment, persons may find it useful to keep a list of frequently misspelled words, especially those personally relevant terms such as names and street addresses, and practice copying them. Ted has his list in a small notebook and uses it as a reference, continually adding and reviewing words. Paula and Ted both learned to say words as they wrote them, slowly sounding out one syllable at a time. Just thinking the words was no longer enough to produce recall of the correct letters; saying and hearing the sound sent more information through additional brain pathways and triggered the retrieval of the letters. When unsure of spelling, Paula often traces the word on the table top with her finger to rehearse writing.

At times, attempts to remember individual letters that form a word cannot be self-generated, and use of an alphabet line may be beneficial. This is simply a strip of paper with alphabet letters written on it. The person scans this line to find which letter to write next. It is important to realize, however, that letter recognition skills must be intact in order for this technique to be successful. (Aphasia can also cause disruption in this ability.) A typewriter or computer keyboard can serve the same purpose. Betty finds her spelling is much faster when she uses her word processor because she can scan the keys and recognize the letters she needs. When Ted uses his word processor, he finds he is more aware of his own errors since he can see his writing clearly printed on the screen. Also, many with spelling problems find a dictionary useful, though Ted notes that this is not an effective tool when he can't remember the first letter of a needed word. If first letters are known, however, the word can be looked up and the correct spelling copied or checked. A spelling dictionary, available in most bookstores, contains word lists in alphabetical order without definitions. This makes location faster with less visual information overloading the brain. New pocket-sized computer spellers now on the market may serve as an excellent resource for some. When first letters are entered on the keyboard a visual display of words beginning with those letters appears, which can be scanned to determine proper spelling. Again, intact word recognition skills must be present for maximum benefit (see appendix, "Aids to Help Writing," for a list of spelling dictionaries and computer spellers). Some word processors or home computer programs correct misspellings automatically and may be useful for those who write often.

Retrieval of vocabulary is also disrupted in writing. We have already reviewed some of the changes in vocabulary expressed verbally; as might be expected these changes also appear in written work. With more severe vocabulary loss, even simple words are not easily retrieved, which might make a task like writing a grocery list very difficult and time-consuming. In milder cases of aphasia, only more advanced vocabulary words become difficult to remember.

Because of this reduction in vocabulary, the content of narrative writing reflects less variety, causing many aphasic persons to complain that their written messages sound elementary to them. Tom practiced copying words for two years before he began to develop an ability to retrieve and write simple nouns such as "book" or "car" from memory. Both Carl and Paula find that having someone give them the first letter of the word is useful to help trigger retrieval. At times, they can now scan an alphabet line themselves to trigger recall of other words. In Ted's daily journal he keeps track of words that are difficult to remember, studying them to help expand his vocabulary. A thesaurus may be useful, providing persons with access to a greater variety of terms.

For some, the ability to write words or parts of words will be the most recovery they make in their writing after stroke. Others with milder aphasia may regain capability to write narrative material. This redevelops as an ability to first write short, then longer sentences, and finally to construct paragraphs. Understanding what goes wrong in the multistep process of writing sentences is easier if we examine how it normally progresses.

Let's consider what happens when you want to write a thank-you note for a gift. After getting the paper, card, pen, etc., you sit down and pause a moment before beginning. In your mind, you have an intended message, which you consider and refine, planning what you want to say. Thus a mental outline is created. Next, you focus on your first thought and write it down. After finishing the sentence or series of sentences it took to complete your first thought, you focus on your second thought and begin to write that down, too. You repeat this process until the note is finished. You might pause at times to reconsider the mental outline, or reread a few lines to remind yourself of the next planned thought. If you were interrupted you would probably scan what you had written so far and resume at the place you left off. When finished, you might read the note again to make sure it says what you want. This whole process would operate smoothly on a fairly automatic level. Of course, you weren't born with the ability to perform such an act without thinking about the steps, but years of practice made what you initially learned as a child into a habit. The brain can plan, formulate, retain, focus, sequence, and edit a thank-you note with minimal concentration.

Now let's imagine a person with aphasia facing the same task. He first gathers paper, card, pen, etc.—in itself a difficult task for someone with hand weakness. Or he may have to use the typewriter or word processor when paralysis prohibits handwriting. He sits down with the intended message in mind and begins to plan what he wants to say and how he wants to say it, but the brain injury interferes with this process, making formulation time much slower and creating difficulty getting just the right words in mind. While he concentrates to choose the right word, he forgets the main idea of his first thought because his memory cannot juggle all that information at once. So he writes down the word he has finally retrieved even though it may not be in the order he originally intended. He writes slowly because he is now concentrating on how to spell it. When he is finished, he pauses, uncertain of where to go next. He repeats the word to remind himself of the original idea of his first sentence. If he remembers he then pauses to think, spell, and write the next words using the steps just described. When he reaches the end of his first thought he might try to reread it. If reading problems do not interfere he can look back at what he's written to check it. Since the content of what a person with aphasia writes is impaired in the same ways we discussed in the section on problems with speech, his sentence may have some or all of the following errors: omitted words ("Thank you the pretty vase"), word substitutions ("Thank you for the the pretty dish"), words repeated ("Thank you for the the pretty vase"), misspellings ("Thank you for the pritey vase"), words out of order ("Thank you the vase for pretty"), grammatical mistakes ("Thank you at the pretty vases"), and punctuation errors. Sentence structure is typically simplified, without the more complex clauses and compound sentences we use for flow and variety. As the person with aphasia is rereading his sentence to find his mistakes, his brain does not automatically see errors anymore. If he is to make changes in what he has just written, he must concentrate on finding the mistake, analyze it to see what type of error it is, then determine how to correct it. He has to make these corrections one at a time and therefore must spend an excessive amount of time revising this first sentence to get it to read correctly.

When he is finally done with one sentence, it may be similar to but is no longer exactly like his original idea. Furthermore, it is still likely to have errors he is not aware of since the aphasia has also compromised his ability to scan and read his own writing. Much time has probably elapsed since he first sat down to plan what he wanted to say, and the memory of his mental outline for the card has faded due to his need to focus all his concentration on each step as he performs it. If you are finding it confusing just to read and understand this description, imagine how tedious the process is for the aphasic person to carry out. As he continues he must remember or replan his next thought. With each sentence or idea to be written, the person must go through this entire process again, as the automaticity is gone. The brain can now only plan, formulate, retain, focus, sequence, and edit one step at a time— with intense concentration at each level. It is important to recognize how very fatiguing this process can be; after one or two sentences the writer may have had enough for the day. He may not have the thank-you note ready to mail until a day or two after he started writing.

Tom has found it useful to use his own type of shorthand when he tries to construct sentences. He writes only important words to first get his ideas on paper and out of his head, later expanding the grammar into as complete a sentence as he can write and correcting spelling errors. Since writing is so exhausting, he writes much shorter messages than he used to or purchases cards that already have a printed verse and simply signs his name. Paula must spend a great deal of time editing her sentences to change word order, spelling, and word form. The following is a sample of her writing before she edits: "Put the flower in the pot. Pot in the black soil. Plant food is beautiful and the flower is riddances." Clearly, Paula's intended message is to give information on repotting and caring for a plant. Yet organization of her ideas and the words that communicate them are not quite on target.

Ted's difficulty with sentence structure, syntax, and vocabulary is evident in the following excerpt from his journal:

> Good day, I worked all day. Later it the house was running one mile with my dog. And later in the house. Bob came to the house. We had a good time (friend stroke) people. It was really great that came to the house and relax. We talked okay. Later I did bike in the house and later relax.

Again, it is fairly clear what Ted's intended messages are, yet his sentences are elementary. They are short and choppy, or run-on, lacking sufficient vocabulary for variety and clarification. It is particularly frustrating for Ted, as for all adults with writing problems, to see internal thoughts expressed on paper in such an elementary fashion. Ted is well aware that persons unfamiliar with aphasia may judge him to be uneducated or incompetent after reading his writing.

Bear in mind the laborious process we have discussed thus far for generating a few short sentences and now consider how difficult constructing a long paragraph, letter, or report might be for the aphasic individual. At this level, organizational problems interfere a great deal. Ideas may be out of sequence and may not flow properly to form a theme. Opening or closing sentences may be missing, and papers or letters may appear to either run on or fail to convey the intended point. Ed, an author before his stroke, found he could write pages of narrative material that he thought were communicating his ideas, but in fact they appeared tangential and confusing to someone reading them. Furthermore, he had frequently written poems, such as this one, prior to his stroke:

Values of Growing Older

Time has robbed me of my quickness and my speed.
It has set a slower pace for me to travel by.
As if to compensate, it gave an inner eye
Which looks ahead and back
Far clearer than I ever saw before.
Going slow is worth the price:
It lets me see the little things.
The tiny things which orchestrate
A counterpoint
To the melodies of life.

After his stroke, he continued to express his feelings through poetry but found it far more difficult to capture the necessary vocabulary and rhythm, as illustrated by the following:

> I could not measure time.
> I did not know the day.
> I could not eat or talk.
> I was depressed,
> but you
> created me
> to learn to read.
> And it was the time
> to visit you
> upon the 7th Floor.
> You sat beside me
> and you read out loud to me
> about my Lieutenant who died
> with machine gun fire.
> You held my hand—
> I cried, I sobbed
> even if I was a man.
> You walk with shadows
> to help me live again.

Through much careful planning, concentration, and revision, Ed's poetry continues to improve with time and practice. He hopes once again to be able to publish his work.

As we have seen, then, the demands of a writing task and a person's capability to meet those demands vary. Individual interest in writing varies as well. Some persons with aphasia had little need or use for writing prior to their strokes and thus have little need or interest in redeveloping this skill. Others may find the process too taxing and demanding and prefer to develop other means to compensate. (Conversely, when speech is impaired after stroke but writing is possible, some persons are faced with the need to rely *more* on their writing as a means of communicating.) For those who need writing in daily activities or to return to work there are several strategies that can enhance the process.

Betty finds problems in organization the most frustrating change in her writing. As we have seen, we internally organize our thoughts into a sequence when composing a series of ideas or a series of words into a sentence. Aphasia causes disruption in this sequencing ability; the ideas become jumbled, making it hard to "grab hold" of each in logical order. Betty has learned to use a word processor since her stroke, finding it improves her organization. Once the ideas are on the screen for her to view she can move words around to make the sequence progress logically. Since she has difficulty writing with her non-preferred hand, typing on a keyboard is faster. She can spell words more quickly and thus devote more concentration to planning her ideas. Editing becomes easier as well when she rereads the first draft of her simple sentences and then inserts words to build them into more complex and varied sentences. Once her ideas are typed and can be viewed on the screen, the word processor's editing functions allow her to rearrange the sentence without retyping. Betty now devotes much of her time to writing a newsletter for stroke survivors. With so much practice, her grammatical complexity, variety, and level of vocabulary have all improved dramatically.

Ted also uses a word processor since he can read printed information on a screen much faster. He is able to find and correct his own errors more easily or use a certain dictionary program to have the computer automatically correct his misspellings. Use of a printer allows him to eliminate time-consuming handwriting, making the task much less physically demanding.

Organization can be further enhanced by adding an extra step before writing narrative material. Let's return to our example of writing a thank-you note. Normally, organization of ideas happens internally during the planning stage, before writing has begun. Since this is disrupted in aphasia, the stroke survivor might compensate by organizing ideas on paper, before writing the actual note. Thoughts might be remembered by using key words such as:

dear
thank you
den
pretty
nice
got vase
love Ann

After listing the ideas to be included, the outline can be numbered to arrange logically:

1. dear Joe
4. pretty
2. got vase
5. den

3. thank you
6. nice
7. love, Ann

The outline is now available for review as the person writes the note. He can readily see where to focus his thoughts and devote his energy to forming grammatical sentences instead of struggling to remember his thought. As each idea becomes a sentence, it can be crossed off the list. You can see how outlining can be particularly useful when longer narrative material must be written.

When Paula has an idea she finds it helpful to say it aloud both before and as she is writing. Thus, she can hear herself to see if the message sounds complete, revise the words when necessary, and embed the sentence more firmly in her memory. (Some, like Ed, find it helpful to tape-record the sentence, then write it down as they play the tape back a few times.) Paula also rereads her sentences aloud when editing. Placing a finger under each word as she scans the line helps her detect omitted word endings or errors with verb tense. For final drafts of important information, such as application forms, she has someone proofread them since she is aware she might not find all of her mistakes.

Ed finds rewriting and checking by reading aloud very important in completing a final draft. As a published author, he often used this technique prior to his stroke. He finds he needs to use it more often now. He changes the wording of run-on sentences, alters wording to make sure he is communicating his idea as clearly as possible, and then has his wife reread the material to give him feedback on content and flow.

We often use writing on a daily basis for note-taking. This might occur when we take a phone message, leave instructions for a family member, make a shopping list or "things-to-do list," put a doctor's appointment on the calendar, note directions to get to someone's house, or take notes in class. Whatever the task, we do this to aid our memory and typically do it under time pressure. More than ever the person with aphasia needs to use memory aids. Yet, as we have seen in aphasia, writing is slowed by the extra time needed to retrieve words, spell, or formulate sentences. In addition, it is very demanding for the aphasic person to focus his attention on listening and writing at the same time. It is possible to continue note-taking with aphasia, but certain adjustments are necessary. Tom, for instance, must take phone messages in his job as a pharmacist. Since his right arm remains paralyzed, he must hold the phone under his head with his shoulder and write with his left hand. As this is tiring, he uses a speaker phone instead, freeing his head, shoulder, and arm. It becomes crucial for the aphasic person to ask the speaker to slow down to give him needed extra time to write. Requests for repetition and clarification are also necessary. Use of abbreviations is helpful but this can be very difficult if the aphasia interferes with ability to recall what letters should be used and then what these abbreviations stand for later. In certain situations, such as in a classroom or in a doctor's office, use of these strategies may be impossible; therefore tape-recording what is said provides a permanent record. Later, notes can be taken from the tape. Finally, the person with aphasia can ask the speaker to write the information for him. When Paula needed directions to a friend's house she asked her to write them and draw a map. Those taking classes can also investigate availability of scribe notes or consider arranging for a classmate to provide copies of his notes.

Writing numbers correctly presents another problem with aphasia. Number substitutions, reversals, and omissions are common when persons try to write addresses and phone numbers. Calculation, especially of multiple-step problems or those requiring memory of multiplication and division tables, suddenly seems confusing to most. Betty, for instance, found it difficult to calculate the time needed to cook a roast when she had to multiply total pounds by minutes of cooking time. Ed wasn't able to resume responsibility for balancing the checkbook or keeping track of the household bills for quite some time. It is important to realize that aphasia does not typically cause a loss in the understanding of number concepts, but that naming, writing, and manipulating numbers internally or on paper become harder. Practice with addition, subtraction, multiplication, division, and story problems can help in recovery of this skill. Meanwhile, many find it useful to use a calculator or to rely on others to do the figuring.

Conclusion

In conclusion, bear in mind that a person with aphasia can certainly compensate for functions the brain used to but no longer performs on an automatic basis in writing. To do so, he must first become aware of all the steps normally occurring in the writing process. Next, he must thoroughly analyze his own skills to determine which steps he can accomplish easily, where his strengths are, and where weaknesses are occurring. Then he can develop alternative ways of performing disrupted skills and practice them until the use of new strategies becomes a habit. This is not an easily accomplished goal. It is accomplished with guidance from a speech and language pathologist, who can observe abilities and weaknesses and devise compensatory strategies for them. It is often attainable only after much perseverance over a long period of time and requires an open willingness to change habits ingrained for years. But it can be done. As Tom so often states: "You have to keep pushing—you can never give up."

5.

Psychosocial Issues
Related to Stroke
and Aphasia

While we have discussed treatment centered on the rehabilitation of speech and language and the return of functional skills of daily living, health professionals working in rehabilitation are becoming increasingly aware that an equally important aspect of treatment is education and support of stroke survivors and family as they deal with this illness. In a recent project, Dr. Feibel (1979) and other researchers interviewed eighty-five stroke patients during the six months following their return home from the hospital. They found a high incidence of depression, anger, and anxiety. Equally common were social isolation, reduced community involvement, economic strain, and disruption of normal family functioning. This research emphasizes the importance of looking at these emotional issues; if stroke rehabilitation is to be truly effective, it must address quality of life after the stroke.

Our six families shared thoughts about these important issues, explaining how stroke affected each family member and disclosing that the more they learned about the effects of stroke and long-term disability, the easier it was to move forward in recovery. Becoming aware of just how far-reaching the effects of this illness can be helped them to realize they were not alone and that their reactions were quite normal. They welcomed the opportunity to share insights and new knowledge about this illness with others who now may be facing the same journey to recovery.

Loss and Grief

To begin, we think it essential for everyone involved to understand the process of grief. Grieving occurs with *any* major loss, including a stroke. It is complex, with predictable stages but with an unpredictable duration and intensity of each. People do not grieve in the same way or in the same time frame. Among other factors, the nature and degree of disability as well as the person's age at the time of the stroke will influence grieving. For example, families of younger stroke survivors say grief is more acute because the survivors have forever lost the possibility of what they could have become, never experiencing all that they might have in life. Families of older stroke survivors may be more resigned in their grieving. Many confront, perhaps for the first time, their own mortality. In reality there is no way to measure or compare degrees of loss and grief, but it is important to be aware of exactly what stages everyone will experience during recovery. The understanding of this process can be comforting, since it eliminates a sense of wondering about why certain feelings exist and reassures that such feelings are natural.

While a number of authors have explored loss and grief, the pioneer in this field, Dr. Elizabeth Kubler-Ross (1969) differentiates stages of denial, anger, bargaining, depression, and acceptance. As we review a brief discussion of the significant issues involved in each stage, bear in mind that an individual may experience more than one stage at the same time since each is not neatly delineated. Note that we have also included points we consider particularly relevant to stroke survivors and families.

Denial provides a time for persons to assimilate what has happened and to try to deal with it at their own pace. It can be part of shock—the protective mechanism we experience in reaction to sudden, dramatic change. In and of itself, denial is not a negative emotion; rather, it creates a shield against pain. Yet problems can arise between stroke survivors and families when one or the other remains "stuck" at this stage, or between rehabilitation staff and families when the staff person is anxious for the patient and family to "get on with it." Since the time necessary for denial differs with everyone, those passing through it quickly may become uncomfortable and anxious with those experiencing more gradual resolution.

It is hard to draw the line between productive denial and denial that can be destructive; consequently, those making the judgment need to examine each situation, as well as their own feelings, carefully. As might be expected, many persons have used denial inappropriately as a way to handle life crises even before the stroke. It is important to know if denial was a prior coping mechanism, since this will influence the way stroke survivors and families approach the problems and how those working with them will address the issue. If prolonged denial occurs, all need to be sensitive to the appropriate time to address it; this needs to be handled in a straightforward and tactful manner. While everyone does need to deal realistically with the problem, premature discussion of denial can take away hope. So much of rehabilitation is dependent upon good motivation; to become hopeless is to lose an important driving force.

Euphoria is another aspect of denial often noticed in the early stages of recovery. When euphoria is present, someone with obvious problems does not seem the least bit concerned. This response can be directly due to the brain injury and usually does not last long, yet is often unsettling to those who may be feeling deep concern for all the problems they see.

Anger, the next step in the grief process, is one of the most difficult stages. Even under normal circumstances, anger is often an emotion that evokes a great deal of discomfort, both for the person feeling it and for those around him, as it is often thought of as an emotion we "shouldn't" feel, let alone express. In fact, anger is a normal and appropriate reaction to crisis, and it is quite natural for the stroke survivor to respond to his devastating illness by expressing it. Difficulty can arise when the aphasic person, lacking ability to express his anger verbally, resorts to behavioral expression. It can be bewildering to see a previously quiet person act out anger by swearing, pounding, or throwing. Such projections of anger are not an indication that the family has failed to provide appropriate care. On the other hand, there may be a fine line between normal expression of anger and destructive behavior. Anger that is inappropriate and results in the physical abuse of people and/or property is obviously not acceptable and needs to be addressed.

Family members, as they deal with this crisis, may also feel anger and direct it toward the stroke survivor and/or treatment staff. Once again, it is important for all involved to realize anger directed at them should not be taken personally or seen as a failure of their intervention. Progression through this stage of anger can be smoother if communication remains open and constructive avenues for expression are developed. Withholding and suppressing anger results in intensification of the feelings and can lengthen this stage of grief resolution.

Bargaining, the third stage, is a period when the stroke survivor makes promises to "work hard" in return for the removal of an adverse life event (in this case, the residuals of the stroke). This is usually a period of good motivation for everyone. The typical thought process might be, "If I put everything into my rehabilitation, then I *will* get *all* better!" While this determination is of great value, the patient and family must also understand there are no givens in stroke recovery. Even though encouragement is needed, it is important to bear in mind what the realistically attainable goals are. Bargaining can also become a stage where so much energy is invested in getting better that everyone "burns out." While commitment and motivation to improve are critical, everyone should think about tempering his energies with time for relaxation and enjoyment of the present.

Depression, perhaps the most devastating of all grief stages, occurs when the denial, anger, and bargaining no longer work to make it all better and the extent of the loss must finally be confronted. Though difficult, it is an important stage, for one must feel the full pain of the loss before the healing of acceptance can begin. But a depressed person lacks the commitment and drive so necessary during the arduous task of rehabilitation. When dealing with him, it helps to remember that it is not *your* responsibility to get him through the depression. The family and staff often need to look at their own response to this difficult period, remembering their need to "cheer him up" may be because *they* themselves cannot tolerate the pain. This depressed individual needs to be immersed in and work through his sadness, recognizing that his losses are real and must be acknowledged. Empathetic listening, whereby the depressed person is aware that you have *really* heard him without judging as he expresses his sorrow, is most important. He needs time to express, as best he can, what he is feeling without being placated by others. During this period your touch and warmth can be reassuring. Remember that no one can completely understand the grief and sorrow of another; knowing that there is someone to offer support is what counts. As this stage resolves, a person gradually comes to the realization he alone must manage the loss, taking responsibility for the course of his recovery. (At times a person may fail to work through this realization and he may become locked in depression. We will discuss the effects of depression more fully later in this chapter.)

Acceptance, the final stage, does not represent resignation but the capacity to see a situation realistically, acknowledging and recognizing what one can control and what one cannot. With the resolution of grief, a person after a stroke acknowledges his limitations and can now work more peacefully to achieve the best possible outcome.

Emotional Reactions to Stroke and Aphasia

In a previous chapter we discussed our stroke survivors' early emotional reactions in the hospital and upon coming home. Because anger, distress, depression, and anxiety, seem to be universal after a stroke, we would like to expand on how these four understandable reactions can affect recovery. Because the turmoil of a disrupted life can be so tremendous for stroke survivors and their families, these normal responses often seem exaggerated. In some cases, emotional lability or catastrophic response (wherein a person responds to a situation with an inappropriate or very exaggerated emotional expression) is also present due to extensive brain injury, and it can be nearly impossible to distinguish between the emotional frustration caused by the stroke and a real inability to inhibit extreme rage, distress, tears, or laughter because of damage to the brain.

Extended periods of uncontrolled laughing, crying, or angry outbursts can be alarming, especially if that person did not previously express emotions openly. The best way to handle this emotional display is to briefly acknowledge it and then continue as before while he regains control. It can help to remember these responses are usually most prevalent in the initial period following the stroke—especially when the stroke was severe—and tend to become less frequent over time.

Anger and Distress

When Betty first came home, she remembers having a "very short fuse" as she dealt with the frustrations of moving slowly and learning to use just her left hand. She had trouble controlling her temper and felt guilty for responding in anger to family members who were trying their best to help.

Ted found his continual distress was expressed inappropriately at times. "One night I didn't like what Alice cooked for dinner and I threw my food across the table." He feels this incident resulted from having no outlet for his frustrations over daily struggles with speech and language problems.

We have already mentioned how unprepared Eileen felt when Carl started having temper tantrums. He began to control his anger once again when Eileen simply left the room one evening after he "pounded the table so hard, I thought it would break." Time alone helped him inhibit the reaction so that he and Eileen could communicate without upsetting one another.

Depression

Depression, as we have mentioned, is a common and debilitating emotional response. Ted, Tom, Betty, Carl, Ed, and Paula talked about the times when they felt completely overcome by sorrow for the loss of so many things dear to them.

Ted handled his intense depression by changing his focus away from thoughts about the stroke to an exercise program. While this helped lift his spirits, sadness always seemed to be "just below the surface." On the other hand, Tom simply could not relax for what seemed to be forever. Since he had always laughed a lot, his family found it distressing that he rarely even smiled. That ultimately changed after a vacation in California, when Tom began to move into acceptance of his stroke, realizing it was "just the way it is." Upon his return he was at last able to relax, feeling more peaceful and appreciative for each little moment of time.

Paula's depression was intense when she first faced the possibility of dying in her thirties and then the magnitude of her handicap after surgery, but her previous optimistic, highly motivated personality has returned over time. While she still wrestles with depression and occasionally sees a social worker, she feels tremendous strength from having survived the illness and surgery.

Ed's depression was exacerbated by memories. Since he was worried about his friend dying of cancer just before his stroke, this concern returned and intensified afterwards. His war memories, triggered during his stay in the rehabilitation unit, added depression. It took time for him to deal with all these parameters. Eventually Ed recovered an attitude of strength and motivation, "confronting major setbacks in my life as a challenge."

None of these individuals took medication for depression even though it persisted for long periods in most cases and would at times become intense. Eventually, however, they were able to move on to other emotional stages of recovery. Since stroke survivors are facing a very real loss, controversy exists among physicians about prescribing drugs for depression. Some prefer to see patients work their way out of depression over time as they grieve their losses. In addition, many physicians say that determining the proper medication is more complicated since the cerebral pathology from the stroke makes a positive response to antidepressants more elusive. Furthermore, many patients may be taking several other medications, causing further complications in antidepressant treatment. Nevertheless, current research suggests that the location of the lesion in the brain after a stroke may have a direct bearing on the severity and type of depression one suffers. Thus, in addition to dealing with depression as a normal grief response, there may also be an endogenous (inside the brain) or chemical depression that may need to be controlled with medication. Often a combination of counseling and consultation with a psychiatrist who can also regulate medication may be recommended. Although counseling can be difficult because of the limited communication of the aphasic individual, it should be considered, particularly if the depression becomes severe.

Anxiety

Another emotional reaction to stroke, anxiety, occurs in part because of the complete disruption of established patterns of living. In many cases the ability to manage anxiety is further reduced by the brain injury itself. The stroke survivor's response to his anxiety may take different forms. Many feel helpless as Tom did. With little self-confidence at first, he felt continually anxious as he faced situations that previously he would have handled with ease. These feelings of helplessness are often expressed by demands for attention and a need to control situations and life events with seeming lack of consideration for others' needs. Tom continually interrupted Lee at work with pleas to pick him up from his treatment sessions when he went through a period of anxiety about the possibility of more seizures. This type of response occurs, as it did with Tom, because the individual is unable to reassure and trust himself enough to handle the situation. The seeming egocentricity of stroke survivors is a response to anxiety and may partly result from their need to think constantly about their disability, forgetting, therefore, the social considerations necessary when living with others. Tom was so anxious and self-absorbed that he couldn't consider the importance of Lee's job and the pressure she now was feeling as the sole financial provider for the family.

Anxiety as a response to stroke may also be observed in the stroke survivor's need for constant love and approval from others, for reassurance that he is still a valued member of the family. The urgency of this request may stem from a fear of abandonment—either emotionally or to a nursing facility—because he can no longer care for himself. Julie shared that Ed called her continually when he was away from home, most unlike his pre-stroke behavior. He not only found it important to check *on* her but to check *in* with her, somehow needing confirmation that his immediate world was fine and that he was still an important part of it. Any number of responses to anxiety may be observed; it is often hard to know when to respond to this cry for reassurance and when to step away, letting persons work through the anxiety on their own, thereby helping to reinforce feelings of self-worth and capability to handle their own lives once again.

Coping with Change

Stroke survivors are continually handling change in once-familiar life patterns and their environments. They must learn to get through a day with the residual disabilities from this illness. As they discover their own solutions, they may appear to others to be overly rigid when making decisions, solving problems, or completing activities. Tom, for example, refused to leave home for rehabilitation treatment until his bed was made. He also insisted that his coat *always* be hung up in the closet—a complete reversal of his pre-stroke tendency to toss it in any available chair. Even though it would have been easier for her family if she had stayed with her parents, Paula insisted on living in her own apartment. Ted found he had to adhere to a consistent schedule in order to keep up with his program of continuous exercise, reading, and practice in writing. All needed routines and habits firmly established because so much else in their lives had been disrupted. Although their responses may have seemed exaggerated, they provided Tom, Paula, and Ted with a sense of control over certain aspects of their lives, thereby reducing their sense of internal disorder.

Unfortunately, the brain injury makes adjustment to changes brought about by the stroke even more difficult. Language problems and reduced ability to store and integrate information can also affect logical decision-making and contribute to rigid behavior. Whatever the cause, it is useful to remember that the constant need to handle change is exhausting. Understanding a stroke survivor's reasons for his rigidity can help put it in better perspective.

Family members will also have emotional reactions as they face the dramatic changes in their own lives. Feelings may range from sadness and fear over the possibility of more loss to anger and resentment about the stroke itself and finally to guilt about having such feelings. All are normal responses; finding ways to express them can ease anxiety and promote healing.

Dealing with Dependency

Tom, Ted, Paula, Ed, Carl, and Betty talked about loss of control over their lives and feelings of vulnerability. Previously independent and responsible adults, each was suddenly cast in a dependent role. To need to ask others for help was new for them. Although uncomfortable at first, each adjusted to the security dependency brought during the acute stages of this illness. With recovery they became aware they had to gradually learn to break this dependency, but to do so meant taking risks. Answering the phone or driving a car, activities they used to do without thinking, unnerved them. Attempting to resume some of these activities and responsibilities again meant a possibility of making mistakes and perhaps looking foolish to themselves and others. In turn, their families were hesitant to let them try something new because of their own fears and uncertainties about their capabilities.

When Ted started running again, his limited reading skills and vision made reading street signs to find his way very difficult. "The first time out, I got lost. I never told anyone because they would be nervous." Instinctively he knew he had to keep taking steps to regain his sense of independence in spite of any uneasiness he felt; in turn, his family had to relax enough to let him do this. Ted and his family compromised; he agreed to carry proper identification so they would not worry when he was away. As Alice remarked so aptly, "I had to let go, realizing Ted could make mistakes. I couldn't take away his dignity."

Setting Goals

During rehabilitation these six individuals became aware that even with maximum effort, gains toward their final goal of recovery happened slowly. Consequently, they found it helpful to break the process into smaller steps by setting some realistic short-term goals. At first they set goals too high, basing their expectations on previous abilities, or too low, because of limited insight into their current capabilities. It helped them to divide aspirations into categories: what they wanted to do socially, to achieve personally, and to acquire as a new skill.

It is often easier to live goals "in our heads," never breaking this "wish list" into realistically attainable small steps. While it may be time-consuming, it is well worth the effort to write out goals, the steps necessary to achieve them, and a timetable to carry out each part. Such structure is particularly important for all family members after a stroke to help persons focus more clearly on where they hope their lives will go from here.

Paula's goals at one point were to feel comfortable going to a restaurant by herself, to be able to wear her leg brace only half a day, and to read for longer time periods. Considering these "next steps" helped her from getting so discouraged at the enormity of the task of recovery. As she achieved each step and was able to celebrate her accomplishment, it was easier to keep on track, stay motivated, and feel her progress.

These individuals found that using skills of relaxation and visualization (the process of seeing yourself moving, reacting, and speaking as you would like to) helped them reach their goals. Because of the continuous energy needed during rehabilitation, learning to relax is very important. Paula meditates as she listens to tapes. She also finds that picturing herself moving gracefully makes her walking with a hemiparesis seem more fluid. Ed watches birds or takes walks to relax; Carl watches old movies. They all realized that without planned relaxation, tension from the continuous push to recover seemed unbearable and made them irritable. After this necessary "time out" they could return to active pursuit of their goals with renewed energy.

Just as you have always considered life priorities, it may now be helpful to reexamine previously established choices. While some may stay the same, others may change. A few may be impossible to fulfill due to the limitations of the disability, but new goals may emerge in the process. As Betty found, "While there have been many losses along the way, there have been gains too that you must remember." Those feeling a sense of resignation because the stroke has reminded them of their own mortality particularly need to consider setting goals. Although "What's the use at my age?" is a normal response to a frightening experience, it can lead to premature withdrawal from the pleasure of living.

Self-Esteem

Loss of self-esteem is yet another component of major illness such as a stroke. Self-concept, for most of us, is based on our perceptions of ourselves as we function and interact in our environment. A person following a stroke and aphasia suddenly looks, moves, and talks differently. If he saw himself as graceful before the stroke, as Paula did, and now moves more awkwardly, he has a changed impression of himself. By the same token, a person whose social contacts depended on his verbal agility finds his self-concept drastically altered. Because he is moving, talking, and interacting in a new way, friends and family may respond to him differently. This "new" person is a stranger to himself and to others. "Who am I now?" becomes an important question.

Psychologist Dr. Jon Geis (1972) elaborates on the stroke survivor's search to feel worthy once again. A person whose previous measurement of worth hinged on his level of productivity, his accomplishments, and his physical appearance now must think about—perhaps for the first time—his intrinsic worth; his value must now be based on who he is, not what he does. This changed self-perception will take time, but Dr. Geis stresses the importance of this adjustment if the stroke survivor is to feel valued and valuable once again.

Tom sensed his own changing attitude as he recovered. Prior to his stroke he always had positive feelings about himself but afterwards sensed he was treated as "not quite an equal" due to his physical and communicative handicap. On one occasion he decided to purchase a car by himself. At the dealership he found he was not treated as a serious customer: "The salesman first ignored me and then was impatient." Tom had had many similar responses before and finally felt enough self-confidence to openly express his anger. This exchange helped him realize that he was still worthy of respect and consideration regardless of his disability. As he says, "first you need to love yourself."

Sexuality

We found our families wanted to talk about changes in sexuality after the stroke. Most were frustrated, sometimes embarrassed, that no one had helped them understand the relationship between disability, self-image, and sexuality. They were relieved to discover that changes in sexual response were common and that it felt better to talk about them, ask questions, and learn about ways to handle changes. After a stroke a combination of physiological, pharmacological, and psychological factors can influence sexual response. With a poor body image because of the hemiparesis, a person might no longer feel he is sexually desirable and start to have problems with sexual performance. He may lose any interest in establishing or continuing sexual relations. This seeming lack of interest may actually be a lack of confidence and a signal that he needs additional support and encouragement from his partner, or it may be a sign of fear that having sexual relations could cause another stroke—an unlikely event. The able-bodied partner may experience some aversion to resuming sexual relations with a person whose behavior and body are different and then feel guilty over such feelings. Yet these feelings are not unusual, and the healthy partner needs help understanding the basis of his reaction. In other instances, an obsessive preoccupation with sexual intercourse, sexual contact, and/or persons or pictures of the opposite sex may occur. This may signal a lack of confidence and need for reassurance about one's sexuality or it can result from the type of brain injury. Disinhibition, or the ability to control feelings, thoughts, or impulses occurs with more severe, diffuse brain injury.

As sexual relations resume, the hemiparesis will cause problems with mobility, so experimenting with positioning is important; the able-bodied partner will now have to do most of the moving. In addition to problems with mobility, the sensory loss (dysesthesia) that is often part of hemiparesis may make touch on the affected side feel different, often producing an adverse reaction or no sensation at all. Many prefer not to be approached on this side. Since touch is so important to sexual response, the possibility of sensory changes should be considered.

In some instances, men may experience problems with impotence and/or premature or retarded ejaculation, and women may not be orgasmic. (Impotence could be the result of medication and should be discussed with a physician.) When intercourse is not possible, one needs to try new ways of touching to insure closeness. Exploring ways to preserve a loving relationship can only happen with honest and open communication between both parties.

During her rehabilitation Paula received limited information about sexual response and positioning with a hemiparesis. She remembers her doctor telling her that the radiation treatment she received would reduce her sex drive. With recovery her sex drive returned, but she found her fatigue from intense rehabilitation and her medications for seizures interfering with her desire; therefore, sexual relations were more satisfying in the morning. She needed to find new positions for intercourse and found lying on her weak side best. On her back her paralyzed arm would become spastic and get in the way. She was able to resolve this by putting her right arm around her partner's back, holding it with her left hand. Paula also learned she needed her partner to do most of the moving, and he inserts her diaphragm for her. Although sexual relations were awkward at first, she found a lot of experimentation worked to get the most comfortable position. "That can be fun too!" Paula found her ability to laugh valuable for relieving the tension and gradually became able to relax and enjoy the experience.

As her self-confidence has increased, Paula has found it easier to seek activities in her community where she might meet single men. Losing her speech was especially difficult since so much of dating depends on subtleties in communication. At first limited in both speech and mobility, Paula did not feel sexually attractive. She finds establishing a loving relationship to be a great challenge with aphasia and now feels more comfortable when she dates another disabled individual since there is mutual understanding of circumstances. She remembers her reactions long ago when a disabled man approached her for a date. Although she was impressed with this man's self-confidence, she would not have considered dating him because of his disability. Her own disability years later has changed her attitude to one of understanding and compassion.

Sexual relationships also changed for the married couples. Lee "felt more like a mother/caretaker at first, which made it hard to relate to Tom as a wife." Tom was fatigued and depressed from challenges faced during rehabilitation and was often not ready to enjoy their sexual relationship as he had before. As his enthusiasm for life returned so did his sexual desire. Fatigue is still a problem and their sexual relationship is not the same as before, but their life as a couple is improving as verbal and physical communication increase.

Ted's sexual response changed following his stroke in spite of the fact he had no hemiparesis and was not on medication. Now, four years later, he finds his sexual relationship with Alice remains changed even though they continue to have a loving relationship based on mutual caring and respect. Alice wonders if this might be due to changing roles that evolved following the stroke, when she assumed the major decision-making responsibilities, or because of Ted's underlying depression. They have not sought any sexual counseling but have considered the possibility.

Eileen and Julie added that although the sexual relationship has changed in both marriages, they have found new importance in touching. Expressions of tenderness, affection, and kissing have helped to keep the intimacy so important to any marital relationship.

Social Supports

Virtually everyone felt socially isolated after the stroke. Friends, who were supportive during the initial illness, seemed to drift away. Lee and Julie found it helped to educate others about stroke and aphasia, for just as they had learned the nature of the communication problem over time, relatives and friends also had to have time to adjust to this familiar but "new" person. When friends understood more clearly what they were dealing with, they felt more comfortable spending time with Tom and Ed.

Many friendships, however, have been formed on the basis of a common shared activity; when this can no longer be shared, the friendship may wane. Tom and Paula found that since they were in their thirties at the onset of their illness, friends their own age simply had trouble seeing them. This was often the first time they had been in contact with stroke; it was too frightening to comprehend—and most had other concerns besides dealing with serious illness. Betty too felt isolated at first without the shared activities of golf and work; her friends also drifted away. She now finds support and a common bond with others who have had a stroke.

Following the stroke, it may be necessary to reassess the nature of the support system outside the immediate family. If social life revolved around work friendships, as Betty's did, a substitute may have to be found for that important social outlet. At this time of crisis, support may come from unexpected and new places if one can open to the possibilities. Think about any interests that have not as yet been developed and find people with whom to share those unexplored interests. Paula, Tom, and Ed, for example, revived their interest in art, eventually finding ways to share this creative expression with others. Understanding and responding to new needs helps avoid the social isolation so common after stoke. As Betty said, "The bumps of life need the shock absorbers of friendship."

Changing Roles within the Family

Each family agreed they had to make changes in their ways of relating to one another. Some adjustments were a result of new emotions, but many were because established roles now had to be different. Alice and Lee, for instance, became sole financial supporters of their families for a while.

Dr. Susan Wiley (1983) has looked at this "role disintegration" following a stroke. She sees repeatedly that the traditional role of each family member changes. A spouse who had previously stayed home may have to work while the former breadwinner assumes the home chores. A child still at home at the time of the stroke may need to assume new responsibilities. While at times everyone might be willing to make these changes, especially when there is no alternative, some might feel helpless as they see old familiar patterns of relating suddenly shift.

Ted was frustrated that he could not be the main breadwinner when Alice returned to work. He told his son, Sid, that he "just wasn't a good father" anymore since he equated "good" with a father who provides financially for his family. In turn, Alice felt her own sense of helplessness over her circumstances. Having to rely on the financial assistance of her parents "made me feel more like a child than a responsible adult" as she struggled to cope with the "conditions" attached to the gift. Being the sole financial supporter was a difficult role to assume along with being the mother to four children still at home.

Dr. Wiley believes that family members need not be defeated by these sudden role changes but can use this opportunity to grow as a family. Although families are really always changing, the directions in which they move are usually by choice; when a stroke happens, change is determined by necessity. Some degree of choice is still possible; when the family can take a close look at how they live together, they can explore alternative ways of doing things. If needed, intervention by a trained professional can teach problem-solving skills so that this crisis can be viewed as an opportunity for new and continuing growth.

Children's Response to Stroke

Like adults, children will differ in their reaction to the situation following a stroke. Depending on the age, maturity, and personality of the child, responses can range from withdrawal to a ready assumption of new responsibilities. Whatever the response, the abrupt change in their environment is a real threat to children's sense of security. Because children might feel they cannot discuss or really don't fully understand the wide range of feelings they are experiencing and the implications of this illness, they may be hesitant to talk with an already overburdened parent. It becomes especially important then that opportunities for expression are made available.

The Martin siblings differed in their response to their dad's stroke; Stacey assumed the role of family decision-maker at the age of only thirteen and was the primary mover in pushing her dad to recover. But three years into his recovery, she found she could no longer cope herself; she had a delayed response to her loss. This began a period of rebellion against added responsibilities and lack of time to spend with her friends. "I realized I had to give up the 'old dad' and get to know this 'new' person." Stacey matured very quickly and sometimes resents that her teen-age years were spent coping with sorrow and more responsibility than she would have wanted. She also knows, however, that she has gained in self-knowledge and shows insight into people and situations well beyond her current seventeen years. In contrast, her brother rebelled outwardly in response to the changes in the family right after the stroke, and Tom finally had to ask his son to leave the house because of the negative effect his behavior was having on the rest of the family. Tom, Jr., now has a friend whose own father had a stroke. He found he was better able to discuss his feelings with someone outside the family. This friend helped him to understand his father's stroke so that Tom now finds his relationship improving. Like many teenagers, rebellion had been his typical response before the stroke, but it added to the family's stress and sorrow when it became even more pronounced during the crisis.

The four Lambert children were all living at home when Ted was sick. Since they had already dealt with serious illness during their dad's open-heart surgery, they were able to draw on some of their survival skills to help get through this new crisis. While each responded differently and has varied memories of this event, they were able to support one another while their parents were unavailable. Sid, as the oldest, assumed responsibilities to help his mother care for the house. Although Alice needed this help, Sid's assumption of the role of confidant and helper to his mother was sometimes hard for Ted. He realized the importance of it but also resented that his son had assumed this role when he himself could not. It is not unusual to find the oldest son or daughter assuming the role of parent—a need perhaps in the acute stage following a stroke but a role that must gradually be relinquished as the stroke survivor is able to assume more responsibility.

Community Resources

Most of our families were interested in resources available in the community or rehabilitation facility. In particular, stroke clubs, counseling, and support groups seemed to offer the most benefits. (For those lacking resources in their area, publications that may add to understanding of stroke and aphasia are listed in the appendix "Information about Stroke and Aphasia.") Julie and Eileen noted that their lack of energy as they dealt with the initial crisis made finding time to seek out and use resources difficult. The extra care required by their husbands prevented them from exploring ways to understand and cope with their current situation as much as they would have liked.

Stroke Clubs

Stroke clubs are usually sponsored by a community recreation department or a local hospital and can offer an opportunity to socialize with others in similar circumstances. Such a club can also provide information about strokes. Paula attended meetings at two different stroke clubs but found most of the members were older. Since the issues raised were not always relevant to her, this was not a good resource. By contrast, Betty's participation in a stroke club was a significant turning point in her healing. She was initially apprehensive about attending the meeting because she was afraid of rejection by the other members. (Betty's reaction is not unusual. Trying a new activity could damage a stroke survivor's already fragile feelings of self-worth; therefore, anything new is easier to avoid.) Today Betty is the club's secretary. Her many creative ideas benefit others recovering from a stroke, and the club gives her an outlet to express her numerous talents.

Counseling

Another resource worth considering, but often overlooked, is counseling for stroke survivors and/or family members. Unresolved family or personal conflicts as well as role changes within a family may require therapeutic intervention. One obvious complication in counseling is the aphasic person's problem with communication. Often, however, a therapist can see a family without involving the stroke survivor. Psychiatrists, social workers, and psychologists are community resources for this service. A psychiatrist is a physician trained to diagnose and treat persons with emotional disorders and can also prescribe drugs that may be necessary to treat these disorders. Psychologists and social workers have postgraduate training in dealing with individuals and families having emotional difficulty. Of utmost importance when selecting a therapist is that you feel comfortable with that individual. Further, since this person will be working through the implications of strokes and aphasia with you, it is important that he also has knowledge of this illness and its effects on the family.

Tom and Lee Martin and their children worked with a psychologist who helped them to understand the role reversals now present and necessary in their family. Tom had always been the head of the family; it was difficult for him to relinquish that role to Lee and hard for their teenagers to know which parent to consult. Without his accustomed parental authority, Tom was constantly reminded of what he had lost. The objectivity of a psychologist helped them to understand this situation and not only to adjust to but also to grow in this new relationship.

Paula saw a psychiatrist who helped her talk about dying after she was told she had an inoperable AVM. She found counseling helped her become more comfortable facing death so that she was able to make a tape-recording of her funeral wishes. Paula needed to discuss her death with her family but they felt acknowledgement of death meant "giving up." She worked with her psychiatrist to help accept illness and death while her family was still in the stage of denying that this loss might occur.

Betty was referred to a social worker who helped her talk about her sorrow; she found herself crying during most of the sessions as she tried to cope with the grief associated with her disability and the loss of her job.

Therapeutic intervention does not provide easy answers. Sometimes there may be no resolution to the myriad of problems connected with long-term disability, but counseling does offer a chance to air thoughts and feelings to help stroke survivors move on in their recovery.

Support Groups

Support groups for stroke survivors and family members can be found in a rehabilitation program or provided in the community. These groups operate on the premise that people with similar problems can help one another. They provide an opportunity to share concerns, gain information, and gently confront one another to encourage growth. Once the acute medical crisis is over, the family will be ready to learn more about strokes and aphasia and what their role will be during rehabilitation.

Support groups for families help others to care for themselves as they deal with disability. A group becomes an outlet to express what may be considered socially unacceptable reactions. Talking about these assorted feelings of frustration, impatience, intolerance, guilt, hostility, and helplessness often relieves some of the anxiety. Family members have also experienced loss and shouldn't feel the stroke survivor's needs outweigh their own. It is important not to neglect their own health as the stress of long-term disability can often lead to illness in other family members. Responses from families to the stroke survivor range from being overly solicitous—not feeling they are doing enough—to ignoring the needs of the disabled person, in the latter case often denying the nature and extent of the illness. Support groups can help families improve their self-understanding to better handle this trauma.

Three of the spouses participated in a support group. Julie chose not to participate because she didn't feel like "rehashing the problems"; she found more value in reading about others in similar circumstances. Lee attended several different group sessions:

> I found that as rehabilitation progressed new concerns would crop up. I needed to learn over again how to deal with the stress of living daily with an aphasic person. Each session gave me a new and much needed perspective. At times I would be relaxed, at others I would be surprised when the same fears and anxieties kept returning.

Alice appreciated the support of a group since talking things out had always been her style; in the group she could feel comfortable knowing other members realized what she was going through and were not judging her responses. "I now have the most trouble always being patient and understanding of Ted's problems. Sometimes I feel like a 'robot' and wish I could forget this ever happened."

A support group for the individual with stroke and aphasia seems to be most helpful after his ability to listen improves enough so he can follow the conversations of others without confusion. A group works when the aphasic individual can communicate either through gesturing, writing, or talking and is not hesitant to do so. This interaction gives him a chance to practice newly acquired communication skills in a protected setting as well as a chance to see how others are handling disability. It offers an opportunity to emerge from the withdrawal so common after a stroke and gives him a chance to feel useful by sharing recovery with others.

For the most part, Tom, Ted, Carl, Betty, and Paula viewed their support group experience as valuable. They agreed that it was reassuring to know there were others experiencing similar problems, and they began socializing among themselves outside the sessions. Tom, even when his communication was the most limited, enjoyed a group since others dealing with stroke and aphasia gave him encouragement to move forward in his recovery. On the contrary, Paula was frustrated with her first group experience because she had "too many problems understanding. I wanted to talk . . . but . . . no way." She dropped out, waited a while, and rejoined when her skills were more developed. Betty could talk but chose only to listen at first, finding it "too hard to discuss personal things. As I was more comfortable, I could talk more about myself." Self-disclosure for most is hard. To a stroke survivor, unsure about who he is now that he talks and moves differently, a group experience, as Betty found, can be initially overwhelming.

Conclusion

And so Tom, Paula, Ted, Carl, Ed. Betty, and their families are learning about stroke and how not only to survive the illness but to become part of life once again. Each family has had to allow time to adjust and the space for each to do this. Rabbi Kushner (1981), in *When Bad Things Happen to Good People,* says that after an inexplicable event, we should not get stuck in "why?" but ask instead, "what next?" Families who not only survive but are concerned about the quality of life after stroke are those who learn to adapt to change in their lives. For living assumes continual change. It is, of course, always more acceptable when you have some control over that change; unfortunately, with stroke and aphasia and other illnesses of this magnitude, that decision is made for us. As we have seen in this chapter, each of these families has felt the grief and the sorrow that is part of this disability but also now understands the necessity of finding ways to adapt. As we conclude our stories, we want to share how these families are responding now and what they are thinking as they look toward the future.

6.

Looking to the Future

"To everything there is a season," and as the healing after stroke occurs there must be movement away from illness and a return to involvement in other parts of one's life. With grief resolution there comes a renewed interest in looking ahead. Each family member, in his own way, has made the journey through several stages—hospitalization, returning home, reestablishing daily routines, and beginning to live once again.

Watching Carl in the hospital parking lot on a blustery, windy, winter morning helped crystalize for us just what this journey might feel like. On that day, with no apparent handicapped parking places available, Carl was forced to park in a spot that must have seemed a million miles away. When he stepped from his car, he reached for his cane, stood up with it securely beside him, and took one step forward before willing his weakened right leg to follow. As the wind threatened his already precarious balance, he was forced to pause momentarily before inching forward once again—still bracing himself against sudden gusts, one step at a time, until he at last reached the building. Watching Carl walk with so many factors conspiring against him, we could not help but reflect on the times during recovery when it might seem much easier to just give up and become a passive bystander in life rather than an active participant. There are those times during rehabilitation when the "wind" catches one off balance so that any forward momentum seems to halt or proceed incredibly slowly. Yet at these times some internal fire keeps burning, just as Carl kept walking on that cold, winter morning— walking slowly and, at times, haltingly, until he reached his final destination.

In the early period of rehabilitation when the crisis is acute, those involved seem to live from moment to moment with no time or energy to think about the future. But as the dust settles and daily patterns are established, new thoughts begin to stir, reflecting a need for change and growth within the individual and the family.

Before concluding the stories of these families, we wanted to reflect on what they are doing and thinking about now. With the sudden onset of illness, their lives were dramatically altered, never to return to former ways of living, looking, and thinking about themselves. What do they now feel like? How have life perspectives changed? They all find that what were once considered important life priorities are different. All of them emphasized, as they have throughout the book, the importance of maintaining a sense of humor. The activities they now pursue, while different from before, give a sense of purpose and accomplishment essential to their sense of well-being.

Ed

Three years after Ed Collins's stroke, day-to-day living has a pattern again. It is a different rhythm, made up of new and old pieces, but he and Julie keep working to iron out the kinks. In fact, as time elapsed after his stroke, they found more than ever that the old roles no longer fit. Ed is redeveloping independence and determination, while Julie has discovered inner strengths and abilities. At times when there is tension as these new roles don't mesh, both remind themselves that time, love, and patience will help them fit the pieces together again.

Communication between them is different. Talking and listening to one another now takes more effort—Ed has to concentrate to comprehend specific information and to organize his thoughts; Julie often has to repeat or simplify messages. Nonetheless, they still have frequent discussions, keeping communication as open as possible.

Julie has become far more independent, pleased to see her own growth. "I have much more confidence in myself, making it possible for me to go ahead and take care of some things Ed used to do before his stroke. Sometimes Ed resents this, but he is aware of the reasons for his feelings." She considers looking to the future an issue of survival: "You have to go on . . . can't stay stuck in grieving." Although she would like to see Ed recover to the point where he can truly enjoy reading, she acknowledges this may never happen. "I keep buying him books . . . and for the first time the other day he finally asked to go to the bookstore together." Julie also encourages him to get the most from life. "Ed has so much to enjoy: grandchildren, our walks . . . when he gets frustrated I remind him to forget about focusing on the negatives." They motivate one another by doing things together—canoeing, camping, and skiing. In spite of all the change, "we are getting back to where we were" in many ways.

Ed's professional life drastically changed after his stroke. When he was medically stable and could resume routines at home, he expressed interest in returning to work in some capacity. During his regular visits to his office he voiced his enthusiasm to department directors. Over time it became apparent that this was not coming to pass. Ed began to feel that he was being put off; that he was not taken seriously; and that he was merely a "bee in the university's bonnet." He acknowledged the residuals of his stroke and aphasia but became frustrated that no one appeared interested in learning with him just what his capabilities and compensations were so he might start teaching again. Julie was particularly frustrated when university staff chose to ignore the issues about his stroke and aphasia rather than openly deal with the problems. In retrospect she feels it has been a case of the "blind leading the blind," in that no one at the university knew how to deal with a staff member having had a stroke. She also feels no one took time to learn about aphasia, either out of fear or a simple unwillingness to do so. In spite of Ed's increasing frustration, he chose to fight for return to his position. Julie worried that his determination to return was an indication he was trying to deny he was any different from before. But although a part of her wanted him to retire, she recognized his concerns and supported his decision.

As months elapsed, Ed heard he could "perhaps" try to teach a class—which never seemed to be put on the schedule. At one point he was asked to pass a physical examination. After completion, he learned the results were only valid for a few weeks and were useless because he was not yet scheduled to teach.

Ultimately Ed got his chance to conduct an introductory class in his field. He prepared by practicing lectures to group organizations; some were successful and others reminded him how hard he had to focus his thoughts to stay on the topic and organize his speeches. Both Ed and Julie were thrilled as the term progressed smoothly. Ed's familiarity with the subject matter after years of teaching helped as he worked with his students. What disturbed him was a lack of staff involvement or help. He remembers staring at a movie projector in class one day, struggling to recall how to run it after it was simply rolled into his room and left.

As of this writing, Ed is finalizing his decision of whether to retire or teach part-time through the university's college of life-long learning. Whatever his decision, the important point is that *he* will be making the choice. Julie continues to support him, although she would like to see Ed leave the stress connected with his job behind. She looks forward to the chance for travel and togetherness retirement would bring and chuckles as she admits, "we would be the first couple in history to increase our income with retirement," due to the limitations of Ed's current disability benefits.

A poignant moment occurred last spring when the university honored Ed with a special party. It was only the fourth such event ever scheduled in the United States and involved speakers of national recognition as well as staff and students. As Ed stood before the group, he was able to smoothly deliver a twenty-minute speech, adding a special moment to a wonderful day.

Ed speaks often of the hobbies he plans to pursue. He has dabbled in painting and wants to take a class. He continues to write poetry and has been documenting a personal account of his illness that he intends to publish for other stroke survivors and families. Frequently he speaks at stroke clubs in the area about the subject of "being ignored." He is supported at these meetings by many others, who identify with feelings of social isolation following stroke and aphasia.

What motivates Ed for the future? Walking, travel, birds, his painting, writing, his wife and grandchildren, staying busy, work. And as he moves onward to a new phase in his life he can cherish the memory that he squarely faced the adversity of his stroke and won.

Betty

Today Betty Dankin is in good health; the lung cancer was detected at an early stage and there has been no recurrence. Betty still has a hemiparesis; she walks with a slight limp and has regained no use of her right arm. Her aphasia now slows her rate of speech and the organization of her thoughts. Many times the frustration is apparent as she talks or writes and can't think of the right word.

Yet six years later, Betty's future mirrors her past, as she is still making "nice things happen to me and for me"—just using different avenues. She has regained control of her life, no longer feeling so helpless and hopeless, and has found new people to meet and new projects to complete. Two years ago Betty bought a computer after deciding to write a newsletter directed to stroke and aphasia survivors. She calls it *New Hope* to represent the way she now feels following her stroke. Currently, she has a mailing list of six hundred and depends on other stroke and aphasia survivors and their families to contribute articles about survival skills. For Betty this is yet another way of sharing recovery from major illness so that she does not feel quite so alone. To date she has written several articles for the newsletter, reflecting on the irony that she had to develop a language problem before realizing she had a flair for expressing herself on paper!

Betty's stroke club has also been an important vehicle to express her creativity. She initiated an annual Handicapped Swimmers' Olympics program with the help of other club members to show the benefits of water exercise in enhancing fitness and increasing flexibility. She also finds time to volunteer at a local hospital's speech and language pathology department. She has learned from this experience that she can do the work, it is just slower than before; she would have a hard time returning to her job because fatigue interferes with her ability to "turn out the work."

Financial resources are a major concern as she looks to the future. Betty received retirement benefits from her company but wonders if it will be enough to see her through her lifetime and to cover any potential major illness that may befall her husband. With her residual hemiparesis, she worries she will not be physically able to care for him, forcing her to find a nursing home. Mostly she chooses not to dwell on the "what ifs" but to think of ways to gain more control over her life. She recently planned and successfully hosted a birthday party for eighty people in celebration of her husband's eightieth birthday. Although this undertaking took a great deal of energy and advance planning, most guests weren't aware of her limitations from the stroke. She could have had someone else do the party but wanted to feel the sense of accomplishment this challenge provided.

What does she see as a next step for her? Perhaps learning to play the organ with her left hand. After meeting an organist willing to show her, Betty is now ready to try. She misses golf and has attempted to play using only her left arm, as she has seen others do, but does not feel comfortable with this just yet. Most of all Betty misses her sewing. Although she has tried, she has trouble manipulating patterns and pinning them on the material with one hand. Not long ago she took her sewing machine out to fix a zipper in her husband's trousers. Feeling proud, she asked him to put them on, only to find the opening was sewn shut! "But the stitching was perfect!" she laughs. Betty continues to give herself new challenges, tempering frustrations with a sense of humor and optimism and the knowledge that indeed she will find a way to face anything else the future brings, just as before.

Ted

Four years have passed since Ted Lambert's emergency surgery. As he reflects on the past and looks to his future, he likes the changes he sees in himself. "It's just too bad it took illness to help me understand." His family also sees differences. He is the same person but much calmer, according to his children. "He laughs more, he's not so serious. He used to be as demanding of us as he was of himself." The children recall not wanting to get in the path of his anger. Now when Ted gets angry, he is able to see the situation from a broader perspective and rarely gets as upset as he once did over trivial matters.

Sid was upset when his dad said he did not feel like a "real" father because he was not providing for his family. "What he is doing now provides such inspiration. What more could you ask of a parent? My dad has taken what life has dealt and made it work for him." While his children say they worry about another serious illness, they feel somewhat in awe of this "new dad," whose drive, determination, and discipline serve as an inspiration to them.

Ted now chooses carefully what he does each day, feeling life is too precious to squander on people or events that create stress or are of no interest to him. Because he has faced two major illnesses, he finds time to visit the elderly in hospitals and nursing homes, for "they need to know someone cares and that they can't give up!" His visits help motivate others as they cope with their own pain. "Before my illness, I never would have considered taking the time for this—now it's a top priority."

Ted's aphasia still affects all areas of communication. At first this communication loss left him with only jargon and an inability to "hear" the errors in his speech. Now, even though speech has improved, he still has trouble remembering the exact words he wants to say. His reading is better in that he can read the newspaper, but he still misses much of the information. Ted spells phonetically; his writing now consists of simple sentences and/or sentence fragments, enough to write a message but limited if he wants to write more detailed information.

Interests have changed. Ted has become absorbed in indoor and outdoor gardening. "I used to laugh at my wife because of all the time she spent with flowers and fixing the garden!" He now runs with the family dog—a pet he used to ignore because he resented all the care and attention she needed. His exercise room at home contains his stationary bike, rowing machine, pictures taken during his various marathons and other sporting events, trophies attesting his successes, and a huge fish aquarium. He enjoys just watching the fish as he exercises or works on his word processor.

Ted now sells electrical services, a job he can handle because it uses his abilities as a salesman and does not require that he remember highly technical terms. His work day is shorter because he gets too fatigued to continue communicating well enough to put in a full day. He laments about some wasted years: "If I knew before what I know now, everything would have turned to gold!" With his new understanding and ability to see life differently, Ted wishes his communication did not limit his choice of employment but let him work at a job where he could implement his ideas.

Ted's accomplishments are no longer confined to work but now include running. He successfully trained for and ran his first marathon exactly one year after his stroke. Since this momentous occasion he has continued to win other competitions in his age group. His outstanding accomplishments were featured in the magazine *Runner's World* not long ago. He talks about his great admiration for people in their seventies who still run and keeps exercising to make sure he will be among them. His phenomenal successes with running prompted him to run in the 1988 Boston Marathon. His own written description for Betty's stroke newsletter following this race reflects his thrill of accomplishment, though it also illustrates the persistent limitations in his writing due to the aphasia:

> The thrill is not just in winning. But in the courage to join in the race. I have four marathons. This was the great thing. The Boston Marathon is the best in the world. 25,000 people run when we started all you can see are people, when you run your really walk to start. The people runners in the world. When you run thousand people are saying your doing great. In Boston are four hills and bad, think about after 16 miles there are a large hills called hills for the heart. The day was cold and shower. I really like day like this but cold was hard. But I'm done. I feel good, I have the best of the world and I did it. By the way I did it 4 hours, 40 minutes.

Ted emphasizes that in spite of his exuberance and positive outlook, "nothing is easy with stroke. It's always hard . . . everything takes longer." He finds even the simplest activity takes extra time to think about, plan, and organize before it is executed. To those who know him Ted outwardly appears energetic, enthusiastic, and fun-loving. Inwardly, when he is with others, he must always be thinking about what he wants to say and how to say it. He must continually think of ways to remember daily plans, always making sure he has understood new information correctly. When he runs, drives, or rides his bike, he is always alert for any new situations and must remember the visual impairment on his right side in order to compensate for it. While he has learned to do things better, there will always be constant reminders of his stroke.

For Alice, Ted's wife, life has returned to a more comfortable routine, and their children have moved on as well. Sid received his master's degree in teaching and has moved to another state to pursue his career. Darrin, too, has changed jobs and moved to another area of the country. Susie has completed her second year of college and has taken a new challenge through her synagogue to teach abroad for a year. While Allen has left home, he still lives close by. Alice now finds other issues take most of her time; the aging and subsequent death of both her and Ted's mothers, her children leaving home, and new career decisions for herself.

Alice likes what she has discovered about herself. She now knows she can handle new responsibilities, though she misses sharing discussions and decision-making with Ted. She frets when friends refer to her as "superwoman" because of the way she handled the crisis of two illnesses. Instead, she would prefer others to see her as someone who has, throughout her life, always done what was needed. True, in recent years she has been called upon more frequently, but in her perception, "I had no choice but to do my best with each circumstance."

Ted still wonders if he could have performed so admirably if the situation had been reversed. This he may never know, but he does realize he and Alice have demonstrated many times they are not afraid to adapt to change. They now look forward to a new way of life together as their children begin their own journeys.

Paula

As Paula Sams participated in one of the final interviews for this book, she pulled off her sock and shoe to show me the new brace she was now wearing for ankle support. As I looked at the simple device, no higher on her leg than midcalf, I was struck by the memory of our first meeting four years ago. Then, she had struggled through the doorway toward a chair, supported both by a walker and a cumbersome metal leg brace. Exhausted, she fell into her seat for an hour of practice in thinking of simple words I described (e.g., "car") and listening intently to interpret simple statements (e.g., "Would you use a phone book to check the spelling of a word?"). Later, she said that she would go home and sleep for the rest of the day after an hour's treatment session. Now, after four years, she related her typical day's schedule: rise by 7:00 AM, eat breakfast in or out, drive to do errands, lunch with family or friends, spend a few hours volunteering at a local hospital or attending local functions related to strokes, dine out, and go to bed by 10:00.

Paula's life is once again her own. Her family sees her as strong and self-motivated. Ted, her brother, thinks rehabilitation has only enhanced her qualities of compassion, warmth, and caring. And Cathy openly expresses admiration: "I think Paula is an exceptional person . . . I don't know how I would have handled her situation had it been me." In spite of past difficulties in their relationship, Cathy looks to their future with hope that the two will spend more time together learning about one another. When asked what her advice to families in similar circumstances might be, she encourages "open communication within the family at all times. Parents spending much time with a younger stroke survivor need to take extra time to question and reassure the other children in the family too. I think kids need to be included in the medical conferences as well, so that they learn what to do." Her older brother agrees, adding that he is still not sure what to expect of Paula in the future. "Is it unrealistic for me to hope she may catch up to where she was in many areas?"

Paula's mother feels anything is possible. She has been amazed at her daughter's ability to maintain positive visions in spite of her circumstances. "I have learned . . . the important things in life. What matters is what's inside. It has taught me to look for the good in people and in life." A few months ago Mrs. Sams made the decision to leave the area, moving permanently to the family's lakeside cottage up north. Her decision did not come easily or without pain and a bit of guilt. "I felt badly, that 'You're certainly not a very good mother,' as if I were deserting my children." But Mrs. Sams realized her own energy reserves were depleted. "I've always been a strong person but I'm probably least strong right now." When the intense role of caretaker eased she began to feel periods of depression and fatigue from the "rush I've been through for a lot of years." She discussed her feelings with Paula, facing a reality within her that "when you are sixty-four you feel you may not have many 'best' years left and if you want to do something else in life you better do it now." In the end, she was surprised to find Paula saw her move as an opportunity for more independence. By letting go, each had opened doors for new growth.

As for Paula, she has been actively thinking of her future for several months. She still worries about finances, planning "in five to ten years" to be working at a new career. As yet career options are undetermined, but she is exploring her abilities in art as a possibility. Recently, she enrolled in a class at a local community college. Since she has a new home computer with word processing, she and her brother plan to write a book about her illness and recovery. Her advice to others? "I wanted to die, but life *does* go on. No matter what, keep working at it . . . Give yourself a chance."

Tom

Four years later, Tom Martin is no longer confined to a wheelchair as he was for two years after his stroke. His future, like his past, will be filled with new challenges. Because of the severity of his stroke, all continue to marvel at how far he has come. In addition to improved communication, he has devised ways to mow his lawn, wash his car, and trim the bushes in his yard—all with the use of only his left arm and hand. "I just can never stop trying and . . . eventually I'll make it. I dislike quitting . . . I will be whole again!"

Recently Tom participated in an aquatics demonstration to show the benefits of water exercise. When asked by the program coordinator how he would get into the pool, he replied, "dive, of course!" This was a very difficult maneuver with a hemiparesis, but no one questioned him. When it was his turn, he laboriously climbed onto the diving board, walking very slowly and methodically to the end. Nervous spectators held their breath as he walked, fearful he could lose his balance. When he reached the end, without a second thought he dove head first into the water. Only later did anyone realize this was Tom's first time on a diving board since his stroke. His response: "Oh, the opportunity was there . . . so I thought . . . why not try it!"

Tom's recovery did not stop at the conclusion of his outpatient treatment. He continues to exercise his arm and leg daily and works relentlessly to improve his speaking, reading, and writing. His right side is still weak but he has learned to walk without a leg brace or a cane. His aphasia and verbal apraxia have improved dramatically, as he was unable to talk at all for the first eighteen months. His speech is slow and labored and he often has trouble finding the words he wants to say. He understands what others are saying unless their communication is too involved or he is too tired to listen. He feels frustrated by his slowed reading but this does not stop him from reading the paper each day; he now writes short messages to his family and notices how his spelling keeps improving.

A goal since his stroke has been to water-ski again. Each summer he tries but so far has only bruises to show for his efforts. The practicality of this goal seems unimportant—what is essential is that it keeps him challenged and reminds him to focus on life, not disability. As he says time and again, "I can do it . . . Just give me time."

Tom has continued to keep his skills as a pharmacist current, initially volunteering at the pharmacy where he is part-owner and now getting paid for his work. Working often means standing on his feet for as long as seven hours at a stretch in spite of his hemiparesis. Nonetheless, at the end of a particularly long and busy day, when he feels unbearably fatigued, something "almost supernatural" seems to keep him going. Tom feels a tremendous sense of pride as he becomes more proficient at work and has recently completed the ultimate challenge—making his brain work for twelve hours in order to take a pharmacy exam for licensure in another state. Tom knows that whether he passes or fails, the ability to concentrate for twelve hours following a stroke and aphasia was a remarkable feat.

Role changes were difficult for everyone in the family, but now Tom and Lee's life as a couple seems more normal, although for a long time there was, as Lee describes, "a continual tug-of-war." A dream of Tom's is to take a vacation with Lee to Mexico, just like a vacation they took right before his stroke. With the children growing up and finances less of a problem, this dream may soon become a reality. Stacey will soon graduate from high school and talks about pursuing a career in a health-related field. Tommy has found a job he enjoys and lives nearby with his grandmother. Tom is relieved as he watches his son's newfound enthusiasm for work, sensing that Tommy has finally found some direction in his life after so much unrest in his teenage years. Many of the problems with his family have lessened for Tommy, and better communication and acceptance have followed.

Soon Tom and Lee will move to another state to start a cleaning business. Having faced this illness head-on, they have decided on a new challenge. Although this new career meant giving up familiarity, they realized their previous way of earning a living was no longer an option. They are enthusiastic about their future and know that whether their plans succeed or fail is of lesser consequence than the courage it has taken to change and move on with their lives.

Carl

Eileen Wilson, Carl's wife, smiles as she's asked about her life now. "I'm more happy and content than I ever thought I could be. Life with Carl is different, but just as fulfilling. He now makes the same bed that I used to have to help him into not so long ago." She smiles and laughs more often these days, secure with a newfound sense of confidence. "I never tried to be strong before . . . I didn't have to. I think if I could have been as strong then [before Carl's stroke] as I am now, we could have had a heck of a better life . . . I think about that a lot, how I would have been more help to Carl."

Eileen is happy with the new patterns in their life. She continues to work full-time, coming home exhausted many days. Work serves as an outlet for both her energy and her need to help others. It has also helped her manage the different paces she and her husband now have, a frequent problem for families adjusting to new patterns after a stroke. While Carl remains fiercely motivated and independent, it takes him longer to do things. "As much as I sit on my hands when I'm around Carl I still want to 'do' for him. It's very hard for me to watch him go so slowly, but when I come home at night after a day of activity I almost come to a screeching halt. I'm content to slow down. If I had to stay home all day I would hover over Carl, which isn't good for his independence. We now have the best of both worlds and we're very close."

When asked about the future, Eileen pauses. She remembers when they made nearly every decision about their "tomorrows" together, but realizes this has not happened since Carl's illness. For her, discussing this book rekindled a desire to begin talks about the future with her husband. She would like to work "a few more years" full-time before cutting back, and she hopes they can afford to travel again, perhaps going on a cruise. Other changes she dreams about, but realizes might be impossible, are: moving to a different home, realizing financial security, and seeing Carl talk more.

Carl's residual communication problems from the stroke include aphasia and apraxia severe enough to limit his speech. To express ideas he uses a combination of gestures, drawings, or written letters supplemented with the few words that come.

He now spends his days taking care of the house, running errands, and attending stroke club or language group sessions. He has picked up the pieces from a life that was drastically different to fit them together in a new shape with priorities that are not the same. He refuses to give up his active participation in and optimistic attitude toward life, volunteering for any activity he can find. Although he would love to work, he has been unable to find a job where verbal communication or physical activity is not paramount. As is true for so many stroke survivors, a wealth of intellectual ability and employment capability is trapped inside a body limited by paralysis and communication loss. All too often available employment options are either not mentally stimulating (e.g., sheltered workshop settings) or fail to accommodate the residual disabilities from a stroke. While many resolve their need to keep active by volunteering, an already overtaxed family would benefit financially from a return to employment.

Carl's children like the changes they see in their father; "I never realized how much patience Dad had. Even though he is still very much in control he seems much less critical." Kristen feels that "Dad still provides us with direction, concurrence, and advice. He is interested in what we are doing with our professional and personal lives and our goals and plans. He is happy we are all successful on our own and mutually independent of one another." They see change in their mother as well. Susan likes the strength she sees developing in Eileen, and Kristen sees her parents as having "reversed roles completely without developing confusing attitudes." Things that appeared critical before Carl's stroke seem much less so. Although the children watched their parents give up an "incredible amount," they also saw them "do what had to be done."

Carl knows he will never stop doing, loving, and laughing. And as Eileen so aptly states: "By *having* to slow down, he now has time to smell the roses."

Conclusion

And so we conclude our story, leaving these families to continue on the journey that began when illness so radically changed their course. In a way we are leaving their stories half-told, for while they have traveled far, there is still much left for them to do and experience. As futures unfold, what was envisioned will become a moment of the present. And, as with all of us, we rattle and bang about in the darkness of our present, doing our best to cope with events and feelings that can never be fully imagined or prepared for. These families time and again emphasized how important it is to maintain an attitude of flexibility and a sense of humor while living that moment of the present.

To write a book about individual responses to strokes and aphasia is, as we came to realize, a huge undertaking. While there are general patterns relating to the size and location of the brain injury, no two aphasias are exactly the same, just as emotional responses to this disability differ. Those selected to tell us their stories shared what Dr. Bernie Siegel (1986) in *Love, Medicine and Miracles* calls the "survivor personality." While his observations concern cancer survivors coming to terms with their disease, his comments are universal for those coping with long-term illness. Dr. Siegel describes this personality as both mature and childlike. Childlike because "aimless playfulness" is enjoyed for its own sake, allowing a person to become totally absorbed by an interest or activity. These are the people who take risks and may make mistakes but are comfortable with themselves. They are highly aware of their surroundings, enjoying other people without the need to pass judgment. They have active imaginations and enjoy daydreaming, knowing this helps keep them mentally fit. When people with "survivor personalities" face illness, Dr. Siegel finds they seek solutions to problems, using the trauma to redirect their lives instead of viewing their difficulty as failure. Each person in this book eventually saw no alternative after his stroke but to change, grow, and learn from his experiences.

Those of you completing this book wondering if you would be able to face illness and disability quite so courageously need to remember that none of us can compare our responses to others'. To compare and perhaps judge ourselves as inadequate will only lead to more frustration. Since all of us respond to sudden, abrupt change in various ways, each reacting and coping as best we know how, we need to make sure we are self-loving, self-accepting, and self-forgiving. Gaging our progress by another's timetable won't work; rather, as these families have demonstrated, moving forward can take different directions.

You can make it by traveling your own pathway as Ed, Ted, Betty, Carl, Tom, Paula, and their families have done—by meeting the moment, planning for the future, and letting go of the need to define yourself only in terms of illness. The road is sometimes straight and sometimes crooked, sometimes gravel and sometimes paved, climbing uphill and gliding down through the darkness of the forest and the brilliance of a sunny meadow. Resist focusing on the ground and instead dare to look at the endless possibility that surrounds you. And as you go, laugh, play, and enjoy living, as you have seen these families learn to do, in the spirit of celebration.

7.

The Author's Personal Experience with Stroke

Beth Pfalzgraf

As Sue and I were nearly halfway into the project of writing this book, I hopped aboard a plane one Wednesday evening to begin a weekend getaway with family at a ski resort in my home state. Little did I realize as I packed my bags that those warm-up suits would become my second skin for the next three weeks in the sterile halls of a hospital miles from home.

It only took seconds for a normal day to change to a crisis when Dad suffered a brain hemorrhage the morning we were to return home. In spite of the number of years I had spent working with stroke survivors and their families, struggling to support, motivate, and understand, I had been an outsider. Peering through the windowpanes was easy. Crossing the threshold was not.

Strokes are not selective. They happen just as often to those who know about them as to those who don't, and apparently the fact that I was writing a book about the subject lent me no immunity, even though I would have liked to believe so.

Early on that Sunday morning I began living the stages Sue and I have written about, and I continue my journey even today. But the road has been a bit different for me because of my knowledge about stroke, brain injury, and aphasia. A few sharp turns and deep ruts have been tough to negotiate, but it has occurred to me time and again that I am not the first to travel this path; many other family members of stroke survivors have professions in health care. Perhaps some of you will relate to my experiences as I share my own story.

Some "stranger within me" moved without thought, making quick decisions and giving directions. Moments before we had found Dad struggling with an excruciating headache and nausea

and we were now in the ambulance headed to the nearest hospital, a painfully long hour's ride away. I wondered about this
"stranger"; I had always assumed I would be paralyzed by the
emotions of the situation if crisis hit my own family.

Part of me recognized the signs of brain hemorrhage at the
very first indication that something was clearly wrong with Dad.
Yet another part of me denied this; the severe headache was a
migraine and the constant nausea and vomiting only flu. Thus
began a wrestling match in my private thoughts—"denial" fight-
ing "acknowledgement"—that was to continue until I had clear
evidence what the problem was. Of course this would all be over
when we reached the hospital, and a smiling Dr. Kildare would
give us aspirin and tell us we could all go home. Meanwhile I kept
glancing to the back of the ambulance every few seconds, asking
Dad, "How are you doing?" in terror that this time he wouldn't
answer back.

From the time of our arrival in emergency through the entire
hospital experience, I felt a strong need to be involved with the
medical staff. While part of this need was due to my personality,
part was also due to the fact that I worked in a hospital every day
with those who had strokes and was used to being a part of the
medical team. So watching Dad's gurney being wheeled away
while I was asked to go to the waiting room felt surprisingly
humiliating. I wanted to wave my arms, get someone's attention,
tell them who I was and why *of course* I should be treated differently. Feeling privately foolish and uncomfortable, I struggled
through the wait to see the doctor.

Thanks to the efficiency of the emergency room staff, the
physician spoke to us within a half-hour of our arrival. When he
told us results of the CT scan, part of me froze. I *knew* what this
meant and I was terrified of the possibilities of danger before us.
In spite of the shock, the wrestling match within me to deny
what was taking place ended. A reality had to be faced, and the
precious energy I had been putting into wondering could now be
redirected toward learning, supporting, and coping. I would have
been drained by worry had no one addressed the issue of diagnosis
early.

In the emergency room it had also been difficult to separate
from Dad, since I was terrified I might not see him alive again.
Logically, I knew that tests needed to be done, but logic was not a
very loud inner voice at that time. In my private thoughts I began
to visualize the next scenes: he would gradually become more

lethargic or incoherent; he would shortly lose consciousness; he would become agitated and his personality would change forever. I hesitated to share this with my sister, feeling that talking might lessen my own anxiety but increase hers. It didn't seem fair to unload all my fears and questions, so I held them inside.

It was particularly helpful that we were permitted to stay at Dad's side from the time his tests were completed until he had to be airlifted to a larger facility. In emergency the staff spoke with us as they worked, explaining the purpose of each procedure. While this did not alleviate our fear, it helped to keep it manageable. Although he was in excruciating pain and would not remember later, Dad was fully conscious and was included in all explanations. The physician held the CT scans over his bed to show us where the bleeding had infiltrated. All of this served to reinforce that this was indeed *real*.

Once transferred to a larger hospital, Dad was admitted to the neurosurgical floor under subarachnoid hemorrhage precautions in order to reduce the probability of another hemorrhage. Simply put, he was to lie as quietly as possible in a darkened room for an undetermined period of time with one family member allowed to visit for five minutes each hour. In his case, physicians thought a cerebral aneurysm had leaked and that the possibility of a second bleed, often fatal, was high. He was to remain on hemorrhage precautions until the following morning, when an angiogram could be performed to identify the exact location of the aneurysm. Once again, this information came from the medical staff quickly, within the first hour of our arrival at the hospital. Hearing the worst was hard, but the staff was encouraging, helping us to maintain hope. Because the staff was direct with us in a caring manner, our anxiety was lessened; we now knew exactly what to do at a time we needed direction.

Playing the waiting game was especially taxing, since the possibility of death should the bleeding start again was very real. My thoughts became circular, encompassing everything from Dad's miraculous return home the following day (denial) to visions of planning his funeral (fantasizing the worst). Our family found solace in talking about our feelings to one another, yet I did not feel comfortable sharing my thoughts of what things could be like if the aneurysm began to bleed again.

Each time I was allowed to visit Dad, I found myself wanting to perform mental status evaluations, and each time the nurses entered his room I had to bite my tongue to keep from asking

173

about blood pressure and medications—"So, how is he *really* doing?" I constantly felt the struggle between my role as a daughter and my identity as a health-care professional. Both were major parts of me but I had never had to "be" both at the same time. Struggling to integrate them, I felt a bit like my own version of Jekyll and Hyde. "Daughter" lent caring, concern, and patience to "health care professional," who in turn helped insulate daughter with focus on fact and data. I *needed* both parts of me to be recognized, needed to talk about this crisis as a daughter and as a health professional so that I could completely work through my fear and loss.

Ordinary and seemingly trivial decisions became impossible to make. At one point my sisters and I were struggling to decide whether, when, and how to send in our sister, who was stationed in Alaska, to see Dad for the first time. Her presence would undoubtedly indicate to him the gravity of the situation, since she was rarely able to make the trip back east. Would the shock of realizing how seriously ill he must be adversely affect him? A nurse responded to our concern by sitting down with us, explaining how to break the news. Her structure and support helped move us out of our struggle. Another nurse on the night shift came to get us from the lounge whenever she went into the room to check Dad's vital signs. She knew this would awaken him and afford us an opportunity to see him. It reduced our conflicts in having to guess when he would be awake, for we needed to see and console him but did not wish to disturb him.

During this early period I found it emotionally impossible to leave the hospital, and I stayed on the same waiting room couch two rooms down the hall from my father's room. Eventually I was ready to venture away, but since I was three hours from any familiar surroundings I felt incredibly linked to the couch in the lounge. It was *mine* and no stranger should dare to sit on it uninvited. I would stake out my claim with coat, empty coffee cups, and the little pillow the nurses had given me. One morning when I returned from Dad's room I found someone sitting too close to my space, and, feeling like a child, I inwardly pouted. Just being able to glance periodically at the door of his room, meaningless as that may seem, proved to be reassuring. Had I been forced to leave the hospital before I was emotionally ready, my anxiety would have been heightened. By staying in a relatively quiet and private space in close proximity, I actually got more rest to renew my energies. Having *some* place of predictability gave me a sense of control and stability at a time when everything was changing.

When the results of the angiogram were available, members of the neurosurgical team met with our family to discuss diagnosis and recommendations. Suddenly there I was in case review wearing my warm-up suit instead of my lab coat, terrified, dreading what I would find out but needing to know. I felt awkward in this family member role, wanting desperately for someone to take me aside and talk to me, using medical terms to answer the questions I wanted to ask. As the physicians explained their recommendations for immediate surgery, they showed us the angiogram and the type of metal device that would be used to clip the cerebral aneurysm, drawing diagrams to illustrate. We appreciated not being rushed or belittled as we struggled to comprehend. Although I clearly didn't want this to be, I had an image of what would happen next and did not have to waste energy imagining.

The morning of surgery arrived in spite of my silent wishes to turn back the clock. Staff shifts changed, people chatted, drank coffee, and ate donuts—mundane morning acts that I found irritating. Couldn't they all see that this was *not* a normal day, but one reserved for quiet respect for our family's crisis? My last visit with Dad before he was wheeled to surgery was particularly difficult, not only because I was scared I might not see him again, but also because I was terrified of *what* I might see. Having seen different degrees of brain injury, I had visions of him in various states flashing through my thoughts. The surgical approach was to be through the right hemisphere; I did not have to worry about postsurgical aphasia, but my images flipped down pages of descriptive material I had so often shared with families and stroke survivors about right-hemisphere brain injury: attention, perception, affect, integration, judgment, and so on. Scared and feeling alone in my knowledge, I called a coworker and found support in her reminder that surgery was not synonymous with residual injury.

During surgery it was least helpful that we had to move our "camp-out quarters" to a large area just inside the main hospital doors filled with rows of plastic multicolored chairs connected together. My absurd thought at one point—that if one stood up the whole row would have to march across the room together— illustrates the impersonal atmosphere of the situation. True, at that moment we were absorbed in egocentricity, but this special cocoon helps protect emotions and preserve energy for coping with whatever is ahead. We would have felt more comfortable in a quiet room away from ringing phones and circulating visitors. Dad's coworkers came to wait with us. They were simply "there": to entertain, to distract, or simply to listen, and their presence helped make our cocoon a safer, softer place.

Less than two hours after the hurdle of life-or-death brain surgery was left behind, we were allowed to visit Dad's bedside in intensive care. Although it hurt to see his swollen head, reddened eye, and obvious discomfort and agitation, relief flooded through me as, incredibly, I saw for myself that he was "okay." There was hope after all. Once again, seeing him as soon as possible after a grueling day of waiting reduced my anxiety. No doctor's word that he was "doing fine" would have sufficed; as a family member I needed to make that judgment for myself. It was the first night I was able to leave the hospital and sleep easily.

After Dad's transfer from the intensive care unit back to the neurosurgical floor, the daughter and health care professional war raged anew. During visits I couldn't help but scrutinize every nuance of his behavior, struggling to gain some objectivity in a situation that was hopelessly subjective. From my work, I knew that mental stimulation was important to recovery, but I was unable to determine where to draw the line. I wanted to fill the entire day with mental challenges and word games. Furthermore, knowing he generally seemed "okay" was not enough anymore—did he have brain injury or not? I wanted desperately to evaluate every possible aspect of language, cognition, perception, and memory so that we could jump right in there and work with any deficient areas. The health care professional saw his sleepiness as "lethargy," his hesitation as "latency." At the same time, I was aware of the absurdity of this idea: *of course* a person recovering from brain surgery needs extra rest, and I certainly could not sit down and engage in an assessment session because of our relationship. We were father and daughter, not client and speech and language pathologist. I was never able to resolve this inner conflict during the hospitalization period, but as time has passed and we have resumed routines, it is no longer an issue. Perhaps I would still feel this conflict if he had suffered permanent change, but Dad was fortunate in that no residual changes occurred after surgery. This was partially due to the fact that it was not necessary to invade brain tissue to reach the aneurysm because of its location and partially due to the lack of severity of the hemorrhage.

For a period of fourteen days following the hemorrhage, doctors had warned us there would be a 40-percent chance of vasospasm (unexplained constriction of arteries), which could lead to a massive stroke and could neither be prevented nor stopped. We seemed to be jumping one hurdle only to find another in the path before us. Because I knew the characteristics of a "massive stroke," my anxiety never lessened after surgery; it simply shifted to new concerns. Each morning I found myself checking his behavior to make sure it was the same or better than the day before. When fluctuations occurred, or Dad was more tired that day, I lost my ability to recognize this as temporary—so often had I reassured families that fluctuation in recovery is normal, yet I panicked, scared that vasospasm was beginning. I remember writing a detailed description one morning of what seemed to be horrible changes in his condition—*this was it*—to attach to Dad's medical chart. Looking back, I realize that the changes were indeed real, but they were miniscule and could have been a result of fatigue alone.

Such a degree of prolonged anxiety became very stressful. I could *feel* the adrenalin in my body. It was hard but helpful that I made myself leave the hospital each day to swim laps (I had exercised several times a week for some time before) and that my sisters and I took time out for dinner together each evening. After the first few nights of stunned conversation it became okay to laugh and talk about other things too. As the days passed we began to feel a special closeness in our support of one another. We marveled at the ease with which we worked together, discovering so many similarities even though we had spent most of our lives miles apart.

Day by day my emotions began to mirror Dad's progress— rising and falling in the space of minutes. If it was a good day I felt energized, a bad day and I was drained. Burnout was common on these days, and my three sisters and I, who were taking shifts with Dad during the day, began to feel more of it within a few days after the surgery. Dad entered a period of time when he would talk with visitors from outside the family and doctors but became silent and sleepy whenever we were alone in the room. We drove ourselves crazy trying to figure out whether this was an indication of some physiological change or an emotional reaction to our barrage of crossword puzzles and word games and state of constant "togetherness." We were grateful when visitors came; we were running out of entertainment ideas, and we knew the company would be more stimulating. Taking a break began to feel more of a relief than a scare, and I found myself irritated with him—only to feel guilty that I could get angry with someone whom I had nearly lost just days before.

Guessing what to do for an incapacitated loved one is a necessary but tremendous emotional responsibility. My sisters and I knew we had to make decisions and readily did so, but we missed the subtle feedback one ordinarily gets about what is helpful and what is not. There were no smiles when we marched in with Oreos and milk, no "thank yous" after a long day on duty. And of course there couldn't be. Dad was not going to rise from his hospital bed to declare: "You all are doing a fine job—keep up the good work." Instinctively we sensed that what we were doing was appropriate; still, like a child, I wanted *someone* to tell me how I was doing, to "kiss the boo-boo" and say it was okay. Support, at this time, needed to come from other sources, from those who were willing to listen without judgment, to put aside personal needs, and to give reassurance or assistance when needed.

Ultimately, we faced our own chapter of "homecoming," and it became time to begin relinquishing the caregiver role. At first it felt absurd to have overprotective thoughts ("you can't walk up the stairs again—you'll trip"; "you can never take another shower—you'll fall and hit your newly fixed head") because I "knew better," but I could now laugh at myself. My sisters and I stayed a day or two at Dad's home to assure ourselves that a routine was established, and then one by one we broke our special cocoon to fly back into the real world.

Without my network of "specialness" about me I was scared: scared to get a middle-of-the-night phone call, scared to go a day or two without talking to someone in the family, and scared because I no longer knew what was happening—no longer had a degree of control over what Dad was doing. It helped cushion the transition to make plans for a weekend trip to visit just two weeks later.

Returning to work was especially difficult. I was supposed to be treating stroke survivors, but my mind kept superimposing Dad's face on the person in my office. "What ifs" bubbled into consciousness throughout the day in spite of my efforts to keep focused on what I was doing. It was impossible to escape from the issues of brain injury, craniotomy, and stroke because I had to spend forty hours a week absorbed with them. Up until then most of my writing for this book had been done at night; I would not work on it again for many weeks.

Dad looked like "Dad" after the swelling, bruising, and red eye faded. But shortly after surgery I yearned to see the smallest of actions that made Dad *act* like "Dad." The absence of subtleties of communication, sense of humor, and initiative as he recovered from brain surgery made him a stranger. Who was this person gazing back when our eyes met? With his return home came a rebirth from somewhere of little pieces of himself. The more the pieces accumulated the more I relaxed, until we had at some point crossed over a line from "too much stranger" to "enough Dad." Yet he *was* different, not because of brain injury, but because of the journey he had been forced to make. I resented the intrusion of the brain hemorrhage into his life and ours and was angry that fate had thrown unpredictability into my nicely controlled routine.

For the first time it touched my soul that my parents were someday going to die. I had dealt with death before, when my younger sister died after an automobile accident, but this was different. At some point in the future the invisible umbrella of parenthood was going to be taken away. No matter that I lived miles away with a life of my own—this event was going to impact in some way, and Dad's brush with death stirred dusty ghosts of unfinished business from childhood. In the months following Dad's brain hemorrhage a major part of my healing has been to reexamine and resolve the issues that arose from it.

There is no ending to my story, although life has returned in many ways to the rhythm it had before, just as it did for the families in this book. My fears are not yet in perspective, but I have found ways to control them. I can go to work and no longer feel overwhelmed by the idea that "it could have been Dad in that chair." Dad is back to the routine of work and life at home, although the emotional "dust" will take more time to settle. And perhaps for all of us in our family the spark of pleasure we have in our love for each other has grown into flame: a flame we nurture carefully, for the winds that steal its glow have touched our lives.

Appendixes

Prescription Drugs

Hypertensive Drugs

Hypertensive drugs are used for the treatment of high blood pressure. *Diuretics* are a family of drugs that work not only in removing excess water in medical situations where that problem exists but also act as antihypertensives. The mechanism that creates the antihypertensive effect is not clear and is a topic of extensive research. The most commonly used drugs in this category include:

Hydrochlorothiazide (Hydrodiuril)
Chlorthalidone (Hygroton)
Furosemide (Lasix)

The centrally acting *Alpha$_2$ agonists* are drugs that lead to increased activity of the neurons that control peripheral blood pressure in the central nervous system. Therefore, when this part of the central nervous system is stimulated, blood pressure drops. The drugs in this category include:

Methyldopa (Aldomet)
Clonidine (Catapres)
Guanabenz (Wytensin)

Beta-adrenergic blocking drugs are drugs that help slow heart rate and cause other physiological changes that lower blood pressure. The drugs in this category include:

Acebutolol (Sectral)
Propranolol (Inderal)
Metoprolol (Lopressor)

Atenolol (Tenormin)
Timolol (Blocadren)
Nadolol (Corgard)
Pindolol (Visken)
Labetalol (Trandate; Normodyne)
Oxprenolol (Trasicor)
Alpha adrenergic blocking agents help control the muscular tone of blood vessels; muscular tone decreases, causing the blood pressure to drop. The drugs in this category include:
Terazosin (Hytin)
Prazosin (Minipress)
Direct vasodilators cause direct relaxation of the smooth muscle of the blood vessels. As the smooth muscles relax, blood pressure drops. The drugs in this category include:
Hydralazine (Apresoline)
Minoxidil (Loniten)
Calcium channel blockers block calcium ions from entering the cells of the smooth muscle of the blood vessels. As the muscle relaxes, the blood pressure is lowered. The drugs in this category include:
Diltiazem (Cardizem)
Nifedipine (Procardia)
Verapamil (Isoptin, Calan)

Anticonvulsant Drugs

Anticonvulsant drugs control seizures that may occur following stroke. (A patient on anticonvulsant medication will have therapeutic blood levels taken at regular intervals to determine the drug's continuing effectiveness.)
Phenobarbital
Phenytoin (Dilantin)
Primidone (Mysoline)
Carbamazepine (Tegretol)
Valproic Acid (Depakene)

Antianxiety Drugs

Antianxiety drugs work to counteract anxiety. They may also be used in combination with anticonvulsant drugs to control seizures.

Diazepam (Valium)
Chlordiazepoxide (Librium)
Clonazepam (Klonopin)
Oxazepam (Serax)
Lorazepam (Ativan)
Prazepam (Centrax)

Antidepressant Drugs

Antidepressants control depression. (A discussion about depression and stroke can be found in Chapter 5.) These drugs, once administered, will take from three to six weeks to counteract depression.

Amitriptyline (Elavil)
Imipramine (Tofranil)
Doxepin (Sinequan)
Amoxapine (Ascendin)
Maprotiline (Ludiomil)
Trazadone (Desyrel)
Trimipramine (Surmontil)
Fluoxetine Hydrochloride (Prozac)

Antipsychotic Drugs

Antipsychotics are often necessary to control the confusion and agitation that may follow stroke.

Chlorpromazine (Thorazine)
Trifluoperazine (Stelazine)
Fluphenazine (Prolixin)
Thioridazine (Mellaril)
Haloperidol (Haldol)
Thiothixene (Navave)

Anticoagulant Drugs

Anticoagulants interfere with the clotting mechanism of the blood and prevent the formation of clots or the extension of existing clots.

Heparin (usually administered for seven to ten days)
Warfarin (Coumadin) (used for long-term therapy; the peak effect is delayed for seven to ten days)

Antiplatelet Drugs

Antiplatelet drugs act to prevent clots formed by platelets in the blood.

    Aspirin
    Dipyridamole (Persantine)
    Sulfinpyrazone (Anturane)

Steroids

Steroids may be used to reduce the amount of fluids that may enter the brain after normal blood flow has been disturbed following stroke and/or craniotomy.

    Dexamethasone (Decadron)

Diagnostic Medical Tests

A familiarity with the diagnostic tools ordered by physicians following stroke may be helpful as you are faced with these new medical procedures.

Various diagnostic imaging devices are used to determine the presence and/or extent of a lesion in the brain following stroke. Two of these procedures are available through the hospital's department of neuroradiology and help by relaying anatomical pictures of the brain. The first, the *CT* or *CAT scan (computerized axial tomography)*, takes pictures of the brain that are presented in cross-sectional slices. The patient is first injected with a dye to enhance the picture of the area under study and then placed in a machine shaped like a cylindrical cone for the actual X ray. This test may be completed upon admission to the hospital to determine any central nervous system (CNS) pathology; however, in the case of a stroke caused by a thrombus or embolus, a CT scan may not show any abnormality for the first few days. A CT scan will be taken again to show the extent and location of the brain lesion.

A more technologically advanced form of diagnostic imaging is *NMRI* or *MRI (nuclear magnetic resonance imaging)*, which has the capacity to relay information about the tiniest body tissue that previously could only be examined by exploratory surgery. This procedure is done without injecting dyes and without exposure to radiation. It works on the principle of magnetism that exists in all matter, including our body cells. The magnetic devices in this machine pick up the needed information and measure and arrange it in useful visual form. The machine can do such complex tasks as localize brain tumors that often would not be detected by a CT scan.

Two other imaging devices that give diagnostic information that is more physiologically than anatomically based are *PET* (*position emission tomography*) and *SPECT* (*single photon emission computerized tomography*), which are used in the hospital's department of nuclear medicine. PET is a more expensive and complex diagnostic tool than SPECT. Both use a newly developed radiotracer, called Isopropyl-Iodoamphetamine (IMP), which improves the brain image but is costly because of the necessity of producing the substance in a nearby cyclotron for immediate use. SPECT's diagnostic information will be less complex and less costly. Information from SPECT is obtained through the use of a rotating gamma camera that sends images to a minicomputer that, like PET, gives information about abnormal cerebral blood flow. Unlike the CT scan, with these imaging devices information about any abnormalities can be obtained immediately.

There are other diagnostic procedures that you may encounter during the course of your hospital stay. An *echocardiogram* uses ultrasound to detect abnormal activity in the chambers of the heart. This procedure can determine the size of the heart chambers and look at the heart valves to detect any thrombus formation that may be present. If thrombi on the ventricle or atrium of the heart embolize into the circulation, they can enter the brain and occlude the blood vessels.

Noninvasive vascular studies of the carotid arteries (real time doppler) also use ultrasound to detect occlusion or ulcerated plaque in the carotid arteries. This procedure is used first to justify a more invasive study, the arteriogram.

The *arteriogram* gives diagnostic information about the condition of the arteries through X-ray pictures produced by arteriography. The arteries are injected with a radio-opaque material to obtain a clear picture.

An *electroencephalogram* (*EEG*) traces electrical activity in the brain. Because of more advanced medical technology, this procedure is not used as extensively as it once was. It is used most often for those experiencing seizures to attempt to define the area of the brain where the seizure arises.

Language Difficulties for the Aphasic Affecting Reading

Passive Voice

A sentence written in the active voice, such as "Sam hit the ball," is easier to interpret than one in the passive voice: "The ball was hit by Sam." It is difficult for the aphasic to determine the relationship between Sam and the ball in the passive construction.

Omitted Words

When words are omitted for brevity and variety, the normally functioning brain will fill in the missing information automatically. In the command "Open the door now," we know the message is directed at us ("*You* open the door now") without further clarification, but the aphasic person might not. He could also fail to realize that "If it is not done today, it will be tomorrow," means that it will be done, or that "Bob is taller than I" means "taller than I (am tall.)"

Inverted Word Order

A sentence with the verb following the subject is easiest for the aphasic to understand. But this occurs less frequently in more advanced writing. Questions, in particular, split the verb and change the order of the words in the sentence, as illustrated by "Where did you put the keys to the car?" or "Did my aunt come on the 5:30 plane?" Often the aphasic person can only interpret these sentences as statements of fact rather than as questions requiring an answer.

Pronouns

Narrative material makes liberal use of pronouns, some relatively easy for the aphasic to remember (he, him, she, her) and others more confusing (its, mine, yours, whoever). Pronouns can cause confusion as the aphasic person attempts to determine the antecedent. In the sentence "Bob did not like Jean's parents when *he* met *them*," a person with aphasia may not understand what is meant by *he* and *them*.

Prepositional Phrases

This construction is used in many statements to add information about the relationship of a noun or pronoun to some other word in the sentence. Changing the preposition can alter the meaning of a sentence. For example: "The doors are open *at* noon" and "The doors are open *until* noon" mean two different things. The aphasic person can easily miss these little words and see only "doors-open-noon"—and drive to the store just as it's closing!

Connectives

Words such as "and," "but," "because," and "as well as" join ideas in a statement. The sentence "The box will hold *as much as* the suitcase" requires the reader to determine the relationship of the box and the suitcase—a difficult task for the aphasic person. In "I am going to the party *because* it will be my last chance to see Sue," an aphasic person may have difficulty sorting out the relationship of the two parts of the sentence.

Plural Nouns

An aphasic person may fail to notice plural markers. In our language, plurals are typically formed by adding an "s" to the root word. Such a slight change is easily missed. Other nouns have irregular forms when plural (e.g., "child" becomes "children" and "category" becomes "categories"). These words may not be recognized in the plural because it changes the way the word looks.

Verb Tense

Verbs express action, changing to show tense—past, present, or future. Auxiliary or "helping" verbs (e.g., *"could have been* eating") may be added to change verb tense. Furthermore, some past tense forms are made by adding "ed" but others change to an entirely new word ("go," "went," "gone"). The person with aphasia has difficulty recognizing these shifts; by the time lengthy verb phrases are decoded, as in "might have been going," the meaning of the sentence may have been lost.

Verb Forms

When a verb is a participle, gerund, or infinitive, verb form becomes more complex. For instance, the verb "plow" can be used several ways. If it is used as an infinitive, the sentence might read, "The farmer has *to plow* his field." When it is used as a gerund, it may read, "*Plowing* the field has caused many hardships for the farmer." If the verb is a participle, the sentence might be, "The farmer, *plowing* his field, was struck by lightning." With aphasia the ability to recognize the ways these verbs change is compromised.

Prefixes and Suffixes

An aphasic reader may be able to decode a base word but get confused when a beginning or ending is added to the word. In the following: "He *dis*obeyed his parents," or "She was told to *re*apply for admission," the prefixes must be interpreted in order to comprehend the sentence correctly. A person with aphasia may simply understand, "He obeyed his parents" and "She applied for admission." Suffixes can be similarly confusing.

Possessives

The possessive apostrophe is a marker easily missed by the aphasic person. In the phrase "grandma's house," wherein two nouns appear together, the person with aphasia has difficulty determining their relationship. Is grandma at a house or does she own it? The difficulty is increased in an example such as "the store's hours," since "hours" is an abstract concept and it is confusing to consider the store "owning" or "possessing" the hours.

Comparatives

Comparisons (e.g., "long," "longer," "longest," or "more capable," "most capable," "less capable") present problems for the person with aphasia. When irregular comparative forms such as "good," "better," and "best" are used, further complication is added. In "The cake is *good* but the pie is *better*," the aphasic person may be unable to determine which is best.

Negatives

Words such as "not," "never," and the contraction "n't" convert a positive message into a negative. Since the person with aphasia frequently misses words, his final interpretation of a negative sentence is often the opposite of the intended meaning.

Reading Materials for the Reader with Aphasia

Doubleday Large Print Home Library, Customer Service, 501 Franklin Ave., Garden City, N.Y. 11530.

New Reader's Press, P.O. Box 131, Syracuse, N.Y. 13210.
> This press publishes a wide variety of adult-oriented reading materials on a less complex reading level, including a weekly newspaper called *News for You* available in A and B editions. The A edition includes the easiest words and sentence constructions, while the B edition is for use as reading improves. Also included with each edition is a quiz that allows the reader to check his comprehension of the news.

New York Times Large Type Weekly, P.O. Box 54206, Boulder, Colo. 80321-4206.
> This paper uses complex sentence structure but is easier to read because of the size of the print.

Programmed Reading for Adults, Sullivan Press, Webster Division, McGraw Hill Book Co., New York, N.Y.
> This series includes eight workbooks for adults with reading problems, starting with comprehension of words and ending with comprehension of sentences and paragraphs. Questions and answers about the material are included in the text.

Reader's Digest Large Print Edition, P.O. Box 241, Mt. Morris, Ill. 61054-9982.

Talking Books

Tapes are available through the National Library Service for the Blind and Physically Handicapped. To find the nearest supplier, contact your local library. Books and magazines on tape and tape recorders will be mailed to you as part of a federally funded program for people with reading disability.

Note: Computer software programs for readers with aphasia are now available at stores that carry educational materials. It is important to note the level of difficulty of each program and to determine if the software is on an adult interest level.

Aids to Help Writing

The following is a selected list of spelling dictionaries available in bookstores. Brief descriptions are included to give an idea of size of print and number of words. Current retail costs range from $2.50 to $9.00.

Dougherty, Margaret, and Julia H. Fitzgerald. *Instant Spelling Dictionary.* 3d ed. Mundelain, Ill.: Career Publishing.
　　lists 25,000 words
　　small size
　　medium-sized print
Ellis, Kaethe. *The Word Book II.* Boston: Houghton Mifflin Co.
　　lists 40,000 words
　　small-sized print
Griffith, Frances. *Barron's: A Pocket Guide to Correct Spelling.* New York: Barron's Educational Series.
　　lists 25,000 words
　　pocket size
　　boldfaced, medium-sized print
Hill-Miller, Katherine C. *The Bantam Instant Spelling Handbook.* New York: Bantam Books.
　　lists 23,000 words
　　paperback
　　small- to medium-sized print
Miller, Shirley. *Webster's New World Speller/Divider.* New York: Prentice Hall Press.
　　lists 33,000 words
　　pocket size with plastic cover
　　small- to medium-sized print

Stein, Jess. *The Random House Basic Speller/Divider.* New York: Ballantine Books.
>   lists 50,000 words
>   paperback
>   small-sized print

Electronic hand-held computer spelling aids recently debuted in the marketplace. Although we have listed few, we anticipate other companies will soon join the market and that technological advances will lead to the addition of other functions. Before you consider a purchase, a visit to a business supply store to try each and find the one most suited to your needs is suggested. Current retail costs range from $50 to $200.

Language Master (Franklin Computer Corp.)
>   lists 80,000 words
>   has a 35,000-word thesaurus
>   measures 7″ × 5″ × 1½″

Spelling Ace (Franklin Computer Corp.)
Word Finder (Selectronics)
>   lists 100,000 words
>   has a 220,000-word thesaurus
>   measures 3″ × 4″ × ¾″

Word Wiz (Franklin Computer Corp.)

Information about Stroke and Aphasia

American Heart Association. 1969. *Aphasia and the Family.* Dallas: American Heart Association.

———. *Gaining Ground.* Quarterly newsletter. Dallas: American Heart Association.

———. 1974. *Stroke: Why Do They Behave That Way?* Dallas: American Heart Association.

Ancowitz, Arthur, M.D. 1979. *What You Should Know about Stroke and Stroke Prevention.* Bethesda, Md.: National Institute of Health.

Beaumont Health and Rehabilitation Center. *New Hope.* Quarterly newsletter. 746 Purdy, Birmingham, Mich. 48009.

Boone, Daniel. 1983. *An Adult Has Aphasia*. Danville, Ill.: Interstate Press.

Brubaker, Susan. 1982. *Sourcebook for Aphasia*. Detroit: Wayne State University Press.

Courage Center. *Stroke Connection*. Newsletter. 3915 Golden Valley Rd., Golden Valley, Minn. 55422

National Stroke Association. *Understanding Speech and Language Problems after Stroke*. Denver: National Stroke Association.

Tanner, Dennis. 1984. *The Family's Guide to Stroke, Head Trauma and Speech Disorders*. Tulsa: MEC.

Wulf, Helen. *A Stroke of Luck*. Quarterly newsletter. 9305 Waterview Rd., Dallas, Tex. 75218.

Organizations Involved with Stroke and Aphasia

American Heart Association, 7320 Greenville Ave., Dallas, Tex. 75231.

American Speech-Language Hearing Association (ASHA), 10801 Rockville Pike, Rockville, Md. 20852, 1–800–638–6868.

Courage Stroke Network, 3915 Golden Valley Rd., Golden Valley, Minn. 55422, 1–800–553–6321.

International Stroke Foundation (M. Prazich, Director), Scottsdale Executive Centre, 7201 E. Camelback Rd., Scottsdale, Ariz., 1–602–947–0421.

National Aphasia Association, P.O. Box 1887, Murray Hill Station, New York, N.Y. 10156–0611.

National Stroke Association, 1420 Ogden St., Denver, Colo. 80218, 1–303–839–1992.

Bibliography

Abramowicz, M. 1984. Drugs for Hypertension. *The Medical Letter* 26 (676): 107–12.

Ahlsio, B. et al. 1984. Disablement and Quality of life after Stroke. *Stroke* 15: 886–90.

Anderson, T., and T. Cole. 1975. Sexual Counseling of the Physically Disabled. *Postgraduate Medicine* 58 (1): 117–23.

Bardach, J. 1969. Group Sessions with Wives of Aphasic Patients. *International Journal of Group Psychotherapy* 19: 361–465.

Barnett, H. et al., eds. 1986. *Stroke: Pathophysiology, Diagnosis, and Management.* New York: Churchill Livingstone.

Benson, F. 1973. Psychiatric Aspects of Aphasia. *British Journal of Psychiatry* 123 (576): 555–56.

Binder, L. 1983. Emotional Problems after Stroke. *Current Concepts of Cerebralvascular Disease* 18: 17–21.

Biorn-Hansen, V. 1957. Social and Emotional Aspects of Aphasia. *Journal of Speech and Hearing Disorders* 27 (1): 53–59.

Bishop, S. B. et al. 1986. Stroke: Morale, Family Functioning, Health Status, and Functional Capacity. *Archives of Physical Medicine and Rehabilitation* 67: 84–87.

Borden, W. 1962. Psychological Aspects of Stroke: Patient and Family. *Annals of Internal Medicine* 57: 689–92.

Bray, P. B. 1977. Reactive Patterns in Families of the Severely Disabled. *Rehabilitation Counseling Bulletin* (March): 236–39.

Broida, H. 1979. *Coping with Stroke.* Boston: College Hill Press.

Brookshire, R. 1975. *An Introduction to Aphasia.* Minneapolis: BRK Publishers.

Brown, J. 1972. *Aphasia, Apraxia and Agnosia.* Springfield, Ill.: Charles C. Thomas.

Chapey, R., ed. 1986. *Language Intervention Strategies in Adult Aphasia.* 2d ed. Baltimore: Williams and Wilkins.

Cole, T. 1975. Sexuality and Physical Disabilities, *Archives of Sexual Behavior* 4 (4): 389–403.

Conine, T., and J. Evans. 1982. Sexual Reactivation of Chronically Ill and Disabled Adults. *Journal of Allied Health* 52: 261–70.

Cooper, I. 1976. *Living with Chronic Neurological Disease.* New York: Norton and Co.

Evans, R., and S. Held. 1984. Evaluation of Family Stroke Education. *International Journal of Rehabilitation Research* 7 (1): 47–51.

Feibel, J. 1979. The Unmet Needs of the Stroke Patient. *Neurology* 29: 592.

Freese, A. 1980. *Stroke: The New Hope and the New Help.* New York: Random House.

Gardner, H. 1974. *The Shattered Mind.* New York: Vintage Books.

Gardner, H., G. Denes, and E. Zurif. 1975. Critical Reading at the Sentence Level in Aphasia. *Cortex* 11: 60–72.

Geis, H. J. 1972. The Problem of Personal Worth in the Physically Disabled Patient. *Rehabilitation Literature* 33 (2): 34–39.

Goldfarb, L. et al. 1986. *Meeting the Challenge of Disability or Chronic Illness— A Family Guide.* Baltimore: Paul H. Brooks Publishing Co.

Henry, D., T. Hill, and B. L. Holman. 1984. Clinical Brain Imaging with IMP and SPECT. *Seminars in Nuclear Medicine* 15 (4): 357–76.

Henry, R. E. et al. 1984. SPECT: A New Direction for Nuclear Medicine. *Arizona Medicine* 41 (6): 398–401.

Hilton, L., and K. Kraetschmer. 1983. International Trends in Aphasia Rehabilitation. *Archives of Physical Medicine and Rehabilitation* 64: 462–67.

Jaffe, J. 1981. The Psychiatrist's Approach to Managing the Aphasic Patient. *Seminars in Speech and Language Hearing* 2 (4): 250–58.

Kaplan, P., and L. Cerullo, eds. 1986. *Stroke Rehabilitation.* Boston: Butterworths.

Kiely, W. F. 1972. Coping with Severe Illness. *Advances in Psychosomatic Medicine* 8: 105–18.

Kinsella, G., and F. Duffy. 1979. Psychosocial Readjustments in the Spouses of Aphasic Patients. *Scandinavian Journal of Rehabilitative Medicine* 11: 129–32.

Klein, R. 1967. Impact of Illness upon Spouse. *Journal of Chronic Disease* 20 (4): 241–48.

Kubler-Ross, E. 1969. *On Death and Dying.* New York: MacMillan and Co.

Kushner, H. 1981. *When Bad Things Happen to Good People.* New York: Summit Books.

Labi, M. 1980. Psychosocial Disability in Physically Restored Long Term Stroke Survivors. *Archives of Physical Medicine and Rehabilitation* 61: 561–65.

Livengood, B., and S. Winkler. 1982. Drug Therapy in Patients with Communication Disorders. Paper presented at *ASHA* Convention, 19 November.

Murphy, R. 1987. *The Body Silent.* New York: Henry Holt and Co.

Robinson, R. 1986. Post-Stroke Mood Disorders. *Hospital Practice* 21: 83–89.

Rolnick, M., and R. Hoops. 1969. Aphasia as Seen by the Aphasic. *Journal of Speech and Hearing Disorders* 34: 48–53.

Rolnick, M., and C. Koski. 1970. An Aphasic Individual's Reaction to His Communication Problems. *Journal of Communication Pathology* 3: 1–6.

Sacks, O. 1984. *A Leg to Stand On.* New York: Harper and Row.

Shellhase, L. J., and F. E. Shellhase. 1972. Role of the Family in Rehabilitation. *Social Casework* 53: 544–50.

Shrey, D. E., J. S. Kiefer, and W. Anthony. 1978. Sexual Adjustment Counseling for Persons with Severe Disabilities: A Skill Based Approach for Rehabilitation Professionals. *Journal of Rehabilitation* 45: 28–33.

Siegel, B. S. 1986. *Love, Medicine and Miracles.* New York: Harper and Row.

Simonton, S. 1984. *The Healing Family.* Toronto: Bantam Books.

Singler, J. 1975. Group Work with Hospitalized Stroke Patients. *Social Casework* 31 (4): 348–54.

Sjogren, K., and A. R. Fugl-Meyer. 1982. Adjustment to Life after Stroke with Special Reference to Sexual Intercourse and Leisure. *Journal of Psychosomatic Research* 26 (4): 409–17.

Tanner, D. 1980. Loss and Grief: Implications for the Speech-Language Pathologist and Audiologist. *Asha* 22 (11): 916–26.

Werner-Beland, J. 1980. *Grief Responses to Long Term Illness and Disability.* Reston, Va.: Reston Publishing Co.

Wiley, S. 1983. Structured Treatment Approach for Families in Crisis. *American Journal of Physical Medicine* 62: 271–85.

）

Index